Novartis Lectures in Gerontology

Vascular Disease in the Older Person

This volume comprises the Proceedings of a Satellite Symposium
of the 1997 World Congress in Gerontology, Adelaide, Australia.
This Satellite Symposium, entitled 'Vascular Disease in the Elderly',
was held in Singapore, prior to the World Congress in Adelaide.
It was chaired by Professor E. G. Lakatta and sponsored by the
Novartis Foundation for Gerontological Research, Basel, Switzerland.

The Novartis Foundation for Gerontological Research Series · Volume 1 · ISSN: 1460-2520

Novartis Lectures in Gerontology

Vascular Disease in the Older Person

Edited by E.G. Lakatta

Laboratory of Cardiovascular Science
Department of Health & Human Sciences
National Institute of Aging
Gerontology Research Center
Baltimore
Maryland, USA

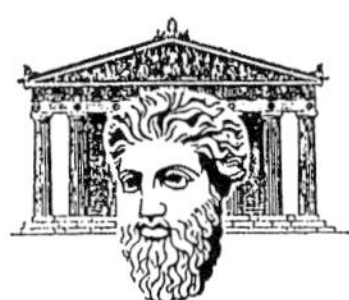

The Parthenon Publishing Group

International Publishers in Medicine, Science & Technology

NEW YORK   LONDON

Library of Congress Cataloging-in-Publication Data
Vascular disease in the older person / edited by E. G. Lakatta.
    p. cm.   —   (Novartis lectures in gerontology) (The Novartis Foundation
for Gerontological Research series. ISSN 1460-2520 : vol. 1)
   Proceedings of a satellite symposium of the 1997 World Congress in
Gerontology, Adelaide, Australia.
   Includes bibliographical references and index.
   ISBN 1-85070-010-9
   1. Cardiovascular diseases in old age—Congresses.   I. Lakatta, E. G.
II. International Congress of Gerontology (1997, Adelaide, S. Aust.)
III. Series.   IV. Series: The Novartis Foundation for Gerontological Research
series, vol. 1.
   [DNLM: 1. Cardiovascular Diseases—in old age—congresses.   WG 120
V331 1997]
RC669.7.V372   1998
618.97'61—DC21
DNLM/DLC   97-41937
for Library of Congress   CIP

British Library Cataloguing in Publication Data
Vascular disease in the older person – (The Novartis Foundation for
Gerontological Research series; v. 1)
1. Blood-vessels – Diseases – Congresses   2. Aged – Diseases – Congresses
I. Lakatta, E. G.   II. Novartis Foundation for Gerontological Research
618.9'7'613
ISBN 1-85070-0109

Published in the USA by
The Parthenon Publishing Group Inc.
One Blue Hill Plaza, PO Box 1564
Pearl River, New York 10965, USA

Published in the UK by
The Parthenon Publishing Group Limited
Casterton Hall, Carnforth,
Lancashire LA6 2LA, UK

Typeset by AMA Graphics Ltd., Preston, Lancashire
Printed by Butler & Tanner Ltd., Frome and London, UK

Contents

List of principal contributors   vii

Welcome Address   1
R. Basdevant

Introduction   7
E. G. Lakatta

1   Coronary heart disease in the elderly: epidemiological aspects   9
P. S. Vokonas and W. B. Kannel

2   Prediction and prevention of coronary disease in the elderly   43
L. A. Simons

3   Cardiovascular diseases and stroke in the Asian population   55
Y. Goto

4   Women, menopause and the primary prevention of cardiovascular disease   73
R. Bonita

5   Non–invasive vascular imaging   91
C. B. Higgins

6   Preventing coronary heart disease: closing the loop   101
E. Leitersdorf

7   To treat or not to treat dyslipidemia in the asymptomatic elderly   105
G. R. Thompson

8   HMG CoA reductase inhibitors: cholesterol lowering for all   117
seasons
J. Shepherd

9   Cost-effectiveness approach to cardiovascular interventions   129
in the elderly
L. H. Beck

Summary   143
E. G. Lakatta

Index   151

List of principal contributors

L. H. Beck
Division of General Internal
    Medicine
PHC 6
Georgetown University Medical
    Center
3800 Reservoir Road, NW
Washington, D.C. 20007
USA

R. Bonita
University Geriatric Unit
Faculty of Medicine and Health
    Science
Private Bag 93-503
University of Auckland
Auckland 9
New Zealand

Y. Goto
Tokai University
School of Medicine
1-2-14 Kugenuma Matsugaoka
Fujisawa Bohseidai, Isehara
Kangaga-City
Kanagawa – Pref.
Japan

C. B. Higgins
University of California
Department of Radiology
MRI Section
505 Parnassus Avenue, Room
    L-308
San Francisco, CA 94143-0628
USA

E. G. Lakatta
Laboratory of Cardiovascular
    Science
Department of Health and Human
    Services, National Institute on
    Aging
Gerontology Research Center
4940 Eastern Avenue
Baltimore, Maryland 21224
USA

E. Leitersdorf
Center for Research, Prevention
    and Treatment of
    Atherosclerosis
Division of Medicine
Hadassah University Hospital
PO Box 12-221
91120 Jerusalem
Israel

J. Shepherd
Department of Pathological
 Biochemistry
Royal Infirmary (University of
 Glasgow)
82-86 Castle Street
Glasgow G4 0SF
UK

L. A. Simons
University of New South Wales
Lipid Department
St Vincents Hospital
Darlinghurst NSW 2010
Australia

G. R. Thompson
MRC Lipoprotein Team
Clinical Sciences Centre
Imperial College School of
 Medicine
Hammersmith Hospital
Du Cane Road
London W12 0NN
UK

P. S. Vokonas and W. B. Kannel
Section of Preventive Medicine
 and Epidemiology
Department of Medicine
Boston Medical Center, and
Boston University School of
 Medicine
Department of Veterans Affairs
 Normative Aging Study
VA Outpatient Clinic
Boston, MA and Framingham
 Heart Study
Framingham, MA
USA

Welcome Address

R. Basdevant
Honorary President, Novartis, France
(President of Sandoz France 1982–1996)

Mr Chairman, ladies and gentlemen, dear friends in medicine and fellow research scientists; as you are all aware, Sandoz and Ciba, two major Pharmaceutical Groups each dating back over 100 years, decided over a year ago to unite forces, and indeed their destiny, by creating a unified group: Novartis. The Latin origin of this corporate name 'novae artes' (in English 'new skills') immediately sets out its strategic focus giving pre-eminence to innovation.

This unforeseen merger between two partners of comparable but complementary strengths has surprised the world's financial centers and has had a considerable impact in the international pharmaceutical industry. The main reasons behind unification were clear. This merger marks the desire of both partners – through the grouping of all their resources and efforts in the fields of life sciences, pharmaceuticals, agriculture and nutrition – to undertake major investments more effectively, and to share the risks of long-term research that constitute innovation. This is the main objective of the new group and a necessity for its future viability within the context of competition exacerbated by the globalization of economic activity. Innovation is undeniably the basis of all major scientific and technological advances and yields the most significant progress, particularly in the field of healthcare. For companies, it is the most robust development platform and sometimes, in extreme cases, the only means of ensuring their survival, thus avoiding social tragedies such as the degradation of unemployment.

This Singapore symposium – the first organized under the aegis of the Novartis Foundation for Gerontological Research – is proof, if proof be necessary, that the objectives of the new group and its commitment to life sciences continue to strengthen the benefit of a partnership with all those who endeavor to promote better health and a better quality of life. It was with this purpose in mind that the Sandoz Foundation for Gerontological

Research was created in 1986; although its activity under this name has now come to an end.

Over a period of a decade, the Sandoz Foundation can pride itself on its achievements. It is indebted first of all to the eminent scientific and medical personalities who put their trust in the organization and gave it their support, and also to the thousands of researchers and participants who have enriched our exchanges through the diversity of their knowledge and experience.

I must also pay tribute to the effective work of my friend, Charles Studer, the Foundation's secretary. His ability, his dedication and his involvement lie at the heart of the Foundation's dynamism. This dynamism can be expressed by means of a few figures. The Foundation's grant of 8 million Swiss francs, approximately 5.5 million US dollars, has been fully utilized, and enabled numerous research projects to be subsidized including the Sandoz prize for Gerontological Research of 50 000 Swiss francs which has been awarded to 18 winners. Furthermore, every two years, the Foundation publishes monographs, so widening the dissemination of knowledge resulting from the Foundation's initiatives. Consequently, it is fair to say that the Sandoz Foundation for Gerontological Research has been one of the key elements leading to a clearer recognition of the health, socioeconomic and human effects related to the extension of life expectancy, not only within the medical fraternity, but also within the media and public bodies.

This awareness on the part of the general public and public bodies, combined with the sharp topicality of the issue, could only encourage the general management of Novartis to pursue its efforts with the same resolve. As a result, the Novartis Foundation for Gerontological Research has taken the initiative in organizing this symposium to establish the commitment of the general management of the new group. I am especially happy to welcome you and to wish you, on behalf of Dr Daniel Vasella, President of Novartis International, a most cordial welcome and many productive exchanges.

As you will see, the Novartis Foundation for Gerontological Research represents a change within continuity. Following on from the Sandoz Foundation, it aims to pursue its mission which I would briefly like to repeat:

> To promote research in gerontology and to contribute to the creation of conditions likely to improve the quality of life of the elderly and their family circle.

Special attention will be paid to the diagnosis and treatment of chronic disorders related to aging, as well as to their prevention, both by means of appropriate medication and more suitably adapted nutrition. These illnesses, about which we should not be fatalistic, are indeed the cause of premature aging and its stigmata.

The Novartis Foundation for Gerontological Research, like its predecessor, plans to award the Novartis prize every two years.

The 'Novartis Lectures in Gerontology', also biennial, should be considered a focal point for multidisciplinary exchanges and a means of continuous education. This is made possible thanks both to expert contributors with authority in the various fields of gerontological research and nutrition in the elderly, and to the publication of monographs, enabling a greater updating of knowledge on the various aspects of aging and the extension of life expectancy.

In her book published in 1996 entitled 'The Revolution of Longevity', Professor Françoise Forette reveals what I allow myself to call her militant convictions concerning the age of retirement and advanced old age. She is currently in charge of the Broca Hospital in Paris and I am pleased to be able to acknowledge both her presence here and her role as a pioneer. She has described the increase in longevity as 'the most important fact of modern times: we age more, in greater numbers, for longer, and above all considerably better'.

The phenomenon is well known to demographers, to gerontologists and, increasingly, to medical practitioners, whose patients aged over 60 sometimes constitute close to two-thirds of their clientele in developed countries. It even surprises specialists because of its extent, its speed, its universality and even its acceleration. Increased longevity represents the greatest demographic upheaval ever recorded, the consequences of which have not yet been completely taken into account, or even envisaged. The age pyramid has lost its traditional shape. Though the Faustian myth of eternal youth remains a dream, man is nonetheless succeeding in pushing back the limits of death. Who among our grandparents would have believed, at the start of this century and even following the First World War, that by the dawn of the year 2000, life expectancy would have leapt by 25 years in nearly all the industrialized countries? It is a gain for a whole generation with, as a bonus, an on-going increase which yields an additional three months every year. The phenomenon persists and lends support to those who predict, in the case of France for example, a further extension of life expectancy of 7 years by the year 2030 and 9 years by the year 2050.

The lengthening of life expectancy in industrialized countries is now mainly due to the reduction in mortality of those aged over 60 years. In the space of 30 years, from 1990 to 2020, their proportion in the population will increase from 30 to 50 per cent in western countries. The generalization of the phenomenon means that it is even more striking in many under-developed countries. In China, for example, those aged over 60 years will be twice as numerous in the year 2020 than they were in 1991; one Chinese citizen out of five will be over 60 years of age. In Singapore, where we now find ourselves, a country often cited as an example of a progressive society, their numbers will almost triple, from 9 to 24 per cent of the population.

The extension of life expectancy, however, should not be an end in itself. The eminent writer and member of the French Academy, Thierry Maulnier, one of the regular participants in the highly popular 'Cross du Figaro' wrote: 'Regular participation in sport means that one does not necessarily live longer, but one certainly lives with more youthfulness'. François Mauriac, Nobel Prize winner in literature and scathing lampoonist, declared with a youthful fighting spirit: 'Despite having one foot in the grave, we should not let someone step on the other one.'

The extension of life expectancy only represents real progress if the quality of life is concomitantly enhanced, together with the exercise of those faculties which dignify man. Medical monitoring and healthcare are essential to prevent and limit infirmities, disabilities and isolation. It is clear that the program for these first 'Novartis Lectures in Gerontology' devoted to 'Cardiovascular diseases in the elderly' has been put together with this in mind. In developed countries these constitute the principal cause of death, in the order of 40 per cent, for those aged 70 and over.

> Three-quarters of those aged over 65 suffer from at least one cardio-vascular illness.

These two facts are sufficient to underline the special interest of this first Novartis symposium, focusing, with good reason, on this very pertinent pathology.

Fortunately the time when the survival of mankind depended upon an imposed, if unjustified, abandonment of the elderly, is long since passed. Great progress has been made, but it can no longer conceal what still needs to be done. There are still, sadly, many people who give aging a debilitating image; this, however, should not negate the millions of elderly people who, generation after generation, age under better circumstances. They are thus testimony to the reality of the quantitative and qualitative improvement in the quality of life. Is there not indeed a fulfilment at each stage of life?

In the pursuit of our efforts, we will be confronted by economic choices necessitated by the need to manage healthcare costs. Thus by way of example, in France, we are still hesitating in putting on the market a prophylactic treatment for osteoporosis – a pathology which nevertheless concerns millions of elderly people. Likewise, some question the validity of stabilizing the mental faculties of patients suffering from Alzheimer's disease if the financial burden for the community is considered too heavy to bear. We all therefore have to remain vigilant and active so that the decisions taken enable us to face up to one of the most stimulating challenges of the third millennium: to simultaneously prolong life itself and to improve the quality of life. This challenge involves each and every one of us. I see it myself, the older we get, the more we are inclined to adopt Picasso's phrase: 'It takes a long time to become young'.

It is the wish that I would like to bestow upon each and every one of you ladies, gentlemen and dear friends. I have no doubt that this symposium will be highly productive and I would like, on behalf of Dr Vasella and myself, to thank the key personalities who have accepted the invitation to preside over and conduct this meeting and especially Professor Sylvester Yong, Chairman of the Congress, and Dr Lakatta, Chairman of Lectures, whom it now gives me great pleasure to call upon.

Thank you for your attention.

Introduction

E. G. Lakatta

The number of older individuals in societies worldwide is increasing rapidly. In many societies the incidence and prevalence of atherosclerotic vascular disease, most notably coronary artery disease (CAD), increase dramatically with advancing age, and although CAD contributes heavily to disability and death throughout life, its impact is greatest in older persons. While the majority of well defined risk factors for CAD remain prevalent in older persons, there is considerable uncertainty about their relative importance. Most notably, an association between high levels of plasma cholesterol and the risk for clinical CAD in older individuals remains controversial owing to several confounding issues.

The definition of the lipid risk factor, apart from defined genetic factors, has rested almost entirely on the measurement of serum lipids. With increasing age, the plasma lipid profile does not match the CAD event occurrence. A blunting of the relative risk of increased plasma lipids in older persons of both genders probably occurs, in part, owing to heterogeneity with respect to health status, the selective removal of those at greatest risk and because age, *per se*, affects the risk for developing CAD, even in the absence of any other risk factors. In other words, age itself is an independent risk factor for the development of CAD. Another source of confusion with respect to the risk of elevated plasma lipids in older individuals is that the medical definition of this risk factor continues to evolve with new data regarding specific lipid subfractions. Because different studies that have addressed the risk of plasma blood lipids have not all measured the same lipid subfractions, or have not included individuals of the same age range, direct comparisons of their results are often precluded. Another source of confusion regarding the risk of plasma lipids is that whereas most observational studies are relatively short lived and focus upon symptomatic, clinical disease, the natural history of CAD usually consists of a prolonged asymptomatic period during which vascular lesions can change dramatically without a clinical event, or change marginally to produce a clinical event.

In addition to the uncertainties concerning the impact of plasma lipid levels on CAD in older persons which arise from the above considerations, information regarding the impact of therapies aimed at plasma lipid reduction in older individuals is far from complete. While numerous, large, well-designed studies published in the last five years have demonstrated dramatic effects of lipid-lowering agents, in particular the hydroxymethyl glutaryl coenzyme A (HMG CoA) reductase inhibitors ('statins'), in the primary and secondary prevention of myocardial infarction and cardiovascular death, these studies have rarely addressed the value of preventive interventions specifically in the elderly. Additionally, research on specific preventive strategies for CAD in older women have lagged behind the focus on the peri-menopausal period, despite the fact that older women are at a greater absolute risk of CAD than pre- or peri-menopausal women. Finally, in the context of scarce resources for healthcare and the enormous growth of the aged population, it is difficult to ascertain whether lowering plasma lipids will provide cost-effective benefits for older individuals in terms of desired health outcomes.

The continued evolution of the saga of the age/lipid interaction in CAD in older persons and strategies for lipid-lowering intervention in persons of advanced age have been re-examined at the *1997 Novartis Lectures in Gerontology*, held in Singapore in August 1997. At this forum, an international panel of experts from the biomedical and socio-economic arenas grappled with multiple facets of the aforementioned perplexing issues. The worldwide magnitude of the CAD problem is addressed by epidemiological comparisons of CAD in western and Asian countries. Differential changing mortality rates among societies and issues relating to gender and menopause are emphasized. Historical perspectives on the definition of the lipid risk factor and its relative potency in advanced age are provided. A critical review of the impact of earlier small intervention trials measuring vascular endpoints, and of more recent larger clinical trials with specific emphasis on clinical outcomes, pinpoints the exact status of our knowledge regarding the effectiveness of interventions in the lowering of plasma lipids. Current studies are described which will, in all likelihood, provide the answers to critical questions regarding lipid screening and treatment in older individuals. Advances in non-invasive methods to directly evaluate the status of vascular lesions are reported. Finally, a summary of the differing public health guidelines adopted by various countries worldwide on whether or not to treat a plasma lipid value in older persons, or even whether to measure plasma lipids in individuals of advanced age, based upon current data of absolute vs. relative risk, primary vs. secondary prevention and cost-effectiveness, is provided.

1

Coronary heart disease in the elderly: epidemiological aspects

P. S. Vokonas and W. B. Kannel

INTRODUCTION

Coronary heart disease is the central component of a broad spectrum of disease conditions affecting the heart and circulation, collectively termed atherosclerotic cardiovascular disease, that progress dramatically as age advances. Although coronary heart disease (CHD) in all its clinical manifestations contributes significantly to disability and death throughout life, its toll is heaviest in the elderly[1-7]. Because there is a substantial paucity of epidemiological information in this area, a detailed evaluation of the role of risk factors for CHD in older persons and the potential benefits of their amelioration would represent an important contribution to the clinical and preventive management of this disease in a large segment of the US and world population.

Considerations regarding the character of CHD and the role of risk factors for its development in older persons, that at the surface may appear straightforward, are in actuality quite complex because, of necessity, they involve interactions of the multiple and overlapping domains of aging, disease and risk factors. This complexity is captured in the form of a Venn diagram proposed by Lakatta and his colleagues[8] (Figure 1).

In this representation, aging denotes the constellation of processes occurring over time in the adult organism, resulting in characteristic alterations of structure and function of body tissues and organs including the heart and blood vessels. CHD represents 'disease' in this context with underlying anatomical and pathophysiological features ultimately manifested as clinical symptoms and complications. Risk factors, in turn, index an array of atherogenic personal traits, as well as lifestyle characteristics including diet and exercise, that are associated with the development of CHD.

"

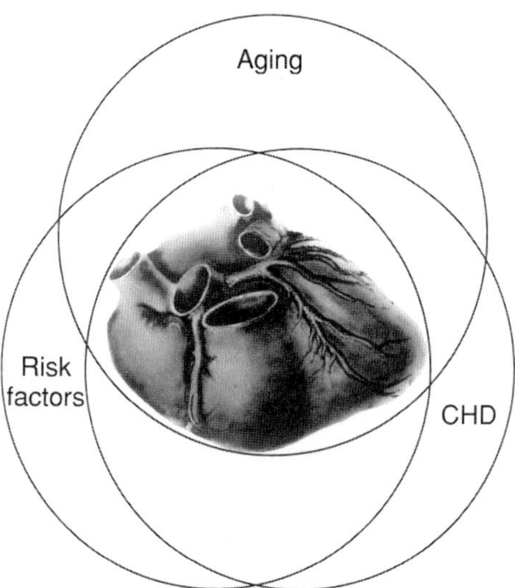

Figure 1 Conceptualized model of interactions between aging, coronary heart disease (CHD) and risk factors for CHD in older persons. Modified after reference 8

Separate perspectives for each interaction among these three domains will constitute the framework for further discussion. First, the relationship of CHD occurrence to advancing age and the character of CHD in older persons will be examined. Next, how established risk factors for CHD change with advancing age and their prevalence in the elderly and finally, the associations between specific risk factors and CHD in the elderly will be discussed, together with available information regarding the efficacy of treating such factors.

Each of these perspectives is systematically examined in 30 year follow-up data from the Framingham Study, focusing on findings in subjects aged 65 to 94 years. Details of the examination and laboratory procedures, response rates and the criteria for disease outcomes in the Framingham Study have been previously described[9].

CORONARY HEART DISEASE IN THE ELDERLY

A fundamental observation of cardiovascular disease epidemiology is the distinct age-related rise in the incidence of nearly all manifestations of heart and circulatory disease across the life span. In addition to CHD, such cardiovascular disease conditions include stroke, peripheral arterial disease and congestive heart failure. The increase in incidence of CHD, however, with advancing age is clearly striking (Figure 2) and illustrates the most important element of the first perspective, the relationship between aging and CHD. Although calculated incidence rates in men and women at far-advanced age are based on relatively small numbers of CHD events, such rates clearly follow trends established earlier in life. Also, while incidence rates in men increase linearly with age, those in women tend to increase more steeply at advanced age approximating an exponential function.

Similar trends of increasing incidence of disease events with age, as noted in Figure 2, are observed in Framingham Study data for both men and women up to age 84 for nearly every major clinical manifestation of CHD including angina pectoris, myocardial infarction, sudden death and death due to CHD[9].

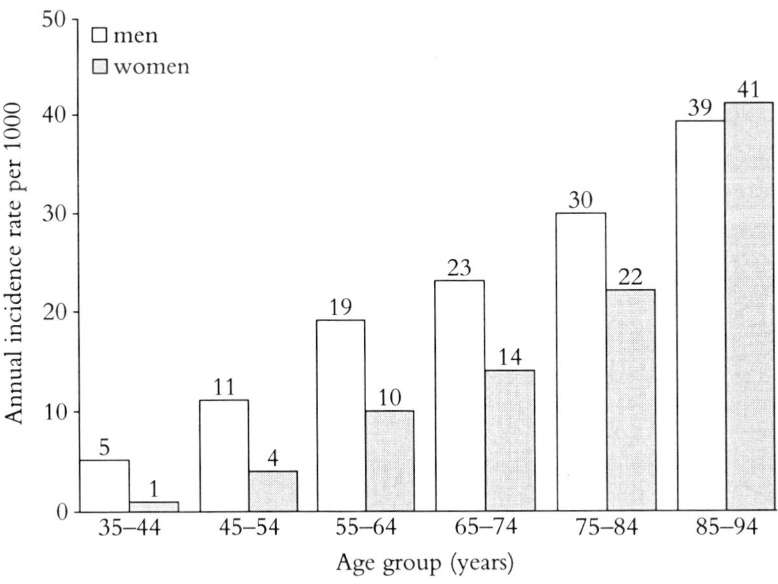

Figure 2 Age trends in total CHD incidence for men and women. The Framingham Study, 30-year follow-up. From reference 3, reproduced by permission

Another important observation regarding the relation of CHD and advancing age is the progressive attenuation of male predominance of disease. This can be discerned by the diminishing differences in incidence rates for CHD between men and women with advancing age (Figure 2) where rates in women exceed those in men at far-advanced age.

The character of CHD according to specified clinical manifestations for older men and women in the Framingham cohort is presented in Table 1. Data indicate the proportion of total coronary events represented by a specific manifestation. Symptomatic categories are not mutually exclusive and percentages exceed 100 per cent because a given subject may have more than one clinical manifestation at the time of their initial presentation within a biennial period. Myocardial infarction represents the most common initial manifestation for CHD in older men, whereas angina pectoris appears to be the most common presenting feature in older women. Angina pectoris in older women frequently occurs as an isolated clinical entity. Angina pectoris in older men, however, is more often associated with acute myocardial infarction, either preceding, or occurring after, the acute event. Coronary insufficiency is the traditional term for unstable angina pectoris referring to the clinical situation of either prolonged chest pain or a progressive increase in the frequency and/or intensity of ischemic chest pain. This manifestation occurs at similar frequencies in older men and women. Sudden death, as an initial manifestation of CHD, occurs somewhat more frequently in older men than women.

A further characteristic of CHD in the elderly is the tendency for a larger proportion of myocardial infarction events to be clinically unrecognized (Table 2). The diagnosis of myocardial infarction in such instances is based on the occurrence of unequivocal electrocardiographic changes consistent with infarction between biennial examinations, where neither the subject

Table 1 Specified clinical manifestations of CHD: men and women aged 65–94 years. The Framingham Study, 30-year follow-up

Manifestation	*Men (%)* (*n* = 244)	*Women (%)* (*n* = 269)
Myocardial infarction	135 (55)	108 (40)
Angina pectoris	73 (30)	123 (45)
Coronary insufficiency	16 (7)	21 (8)
Sudden death	37 (15)	31 (12)

Table 2 Proportion of unrecognized myocardial infarctions by age and sex. The Framingham Study, 30-year follow-up

Age (years)	*Men* %	*Women* %
30–44	29	—
45–54	18	41
55–64	25	31
65–74	25	35
75–84	42	36
85–95	33	46
Average	28	35

nor his/her physician has suspected the diagnosis[10]. Symptoms associated with such events are usually attributed to musculoskeletal chest discomfort, upper gastrointestinal tract upset, gall bladder disease or various other conditions. Approximately one half of such infarctions are completely silent. Unrecognized events represent a large proportion of all infarctions in women, particularly older women.

CHANGES IN CHD RISK FACTORS WITH ADVANCING AGE

Nearly all of the established CHD risk factors change with advancing age. These include changes in blood pressure, serum lipids, cigarette smoking, glucose metabolism, body weight and other factors. Several age-related trends in risk factors and their prevalence in older persons are described below. This constitutes the second perspective of this discussion, the interaction between aging and risk factors.

The most well-characterized change in an established CHD risk factor with age, is elevation of blood pressure. In longitudinal data from the Framingham Study, systolic blood pressure is observed to rise nearly linearly with advancing age in both men and women (Figure 3). Diastolic blood pressure, in contrast, tends to rise throughout middle age in both sexes and actually declines at advanced age. Diastolic blood pressures in women, however, usually remain 5 to 10 mmHg lower than those in men throughout the life span[1].

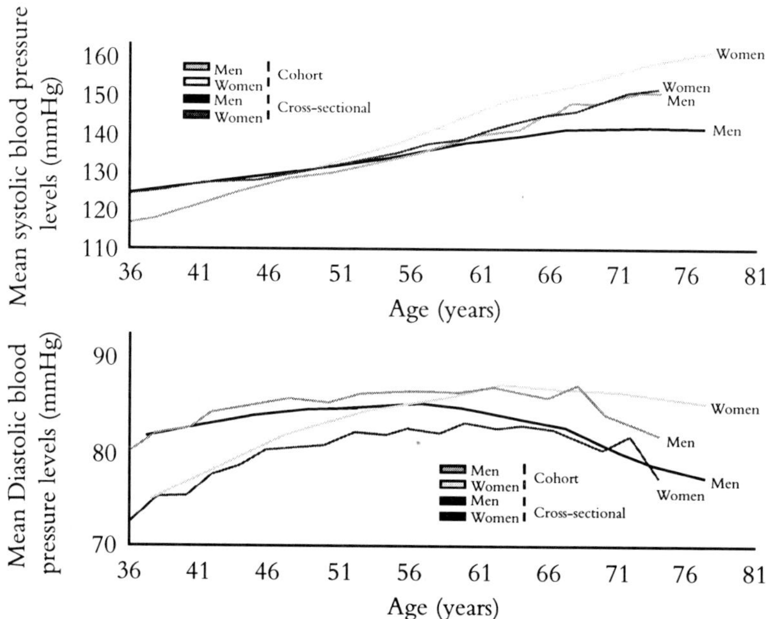

Figure 3 Average age trends in systolic and diastolic blood pressure levels for men and women based on cross-sectional and longitudinal (cohort) data. The Framingham Study, biennial examinations 3–10. Modified after reference 1

The consistent increase in systolic blood pressure is due to progressive vascular stiffening attributable, in turn, to alterations of the physico-chemical properties of the media of the arterial wall including overall thickening and changes in the nature and content of collagen, elastin and possibly other structural proteins that occur with advancing age[11]. This process is dissimilar to that of atherosclerosis which underlies the preponderance of cardio-vascular disease observed in older people.

Although progressive elevation of systolic blood pressure with advancing age is consistently observed in nearly every Western-industrialized popula-tion studied, it does not appear to represent a universal feature of the aging process. Data from a number of isolated primitive populations suggest that this relationship is markedly blunted[12]. Possibilities accounting for differ-ences in age-related change in blood pressure between populations are likely to include genetic factors as well as dietary influences especially the higher intake of salt in industrialized nations[13].

Despite its ubiquity, however, progressive elevation of systolic blood pressure with advancing age should not be construed as an innocuous concomitant of the aging process since it clearly confers increased risk for stroke, CHD and other cardiovascular disease events in both elderly men and women[14]. Elevated diastolic blood pressure also occurs commonly in the elderly and remains an important risk factor for cardiovascular disease, particularly in older men.

As a consequence of the progressive age-related increase, primarily in systolic blood pressure, approximately 40 to 50 per cent of men and women in a typical Westernized population such as Framingham meet one or more of the established criteria for hypertension after the age of 65. For persons categorized as being hypertensive, isolated systolic hypertension (defined as systolic blood pressure > 160 mmHg with diastolic blood pressure ≤ 95 mmHg) accounts for nearly two-thirds of the total prevalence of hypertension in both older men and women[15]. Combined hypertension characterized by abnormal elevations of both systolic and diastolic blood pressures accounts for less than one-third of the total prevalence. Isolated diastolic hypertension is considerably less prevalent in older men and women accounting for less than 15 per cent of the prevalence.

Blood lipids, including serum total cholesterol, also vary with age across the life span and trends appear to be different in women as compared to men. Figure 4 shows cross-sectional and longitudinal trends in average levels of serum cholesterol in the Framingham Study as a function of age. It can be noted that levels in men tend to peak in early middle age and then slowly decline with advancing age. Levels in women peak later in middle age and remain relatively high until advanced age, when a decline occurs. The practical implication of this trend is the relatively high prevalence of hypercholesterolemia likely to be encountered in comparable populations of older women.

Corresponding age trends for specific lipoprotein cholesterol subfractions in the Framingham Study are illustrated in Figure 5. Trends for low density lipoprotein cholesterol (LDL), in general, are similar to those for serum total cholesterol. Mean levels of high density lipoprotein cholesterol (HDL) are consistently higher in women than in men across the age span but tend to decline slightly after menopause. Trends in men remain essentially unchanged throughout life. Mean values of very low density lipoproteins (VLDL) tend to be higher in men than women but trends in both tend to rise throughout middle age and then remain relatively stable thereafter.

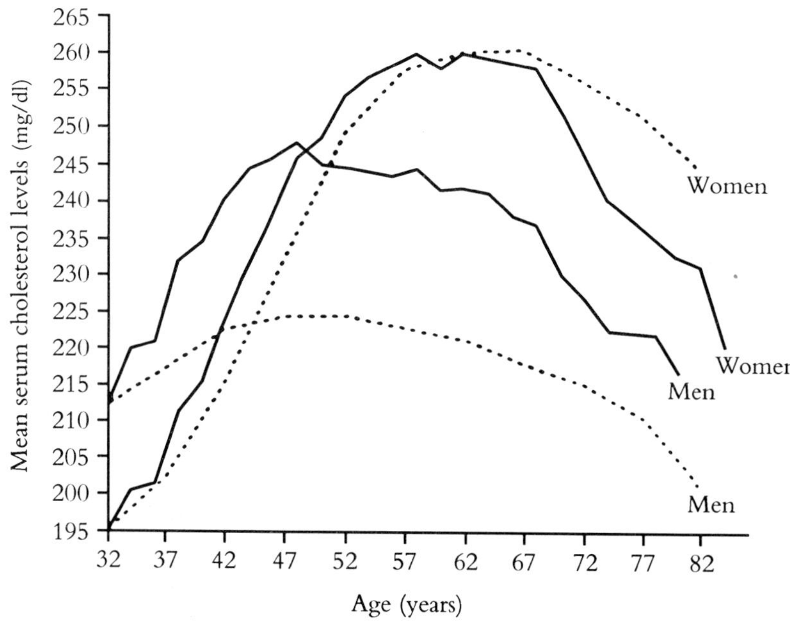

Figure 4 Average age trends in serum cholesterol levels in cross-sectional and longitudinal (cohort) data. The Framingham Study, biennial examinations 1–16. Solid lines, cohort group; broken lines, cross-sectional group

Presumably, these trends reflect fluctuations in body weight occurring at corresponding ages in the sexes.

The prevalence of a number of cardiovascular risk factors in older subjects of the Framingham Study is presented in Table 3. Data are arrayed for each decade of age from 65 to 94 years and separately for men and women.

As would be expected from age-trends observed earlier, hyper-cholesterolemia appears to be quite prevalent in older women. Glucose metabolism becomes progressively impaired with advancing age resulting in increasing prevalence of glucose intolerance in both older men and women[16]. Body weight tends to decrease at far-advanced age. Weight loss, however, represents a reduction primarily in lean body mass, that is, muscle and bone tissue rather than adipose tissue. The result is an alteration of body composition in older persons with higher proportional adiposity per unit of weight[17]. Despite the tendency for lower body weights at advanced age, obesity appears to be well represented in both older men and women in this

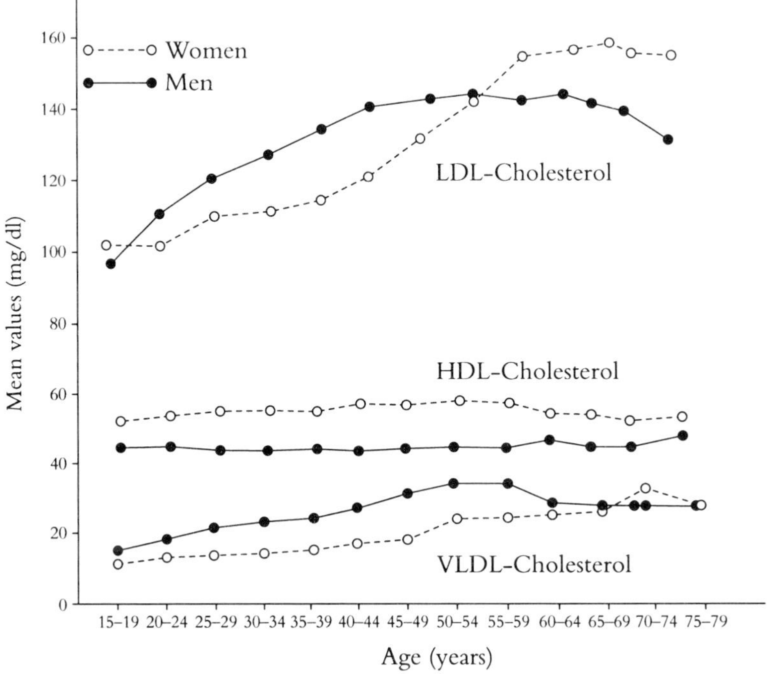

Figure 5 Average age trends in lipoprotein cholesterol subfractions. The Framingham Study, 26-year follow-up

analysis. The prevalence of cigarette smoking appears to decrease with advancing age. This can be attributed not only to higher mortality rates in smokers but also to discontinuation of cigarettes because of health problems or concerns in older persons. The prevalence of left ventricular hypertrophy as determined by the electrocardiogram increases with advancing age in both older men and women.

From the foregoing analysis, it is clear that the majority of established risk factors for CHD in middle-aged persons are prevalent in the elderly. What remains is the task of marshalling evidence to address the question whether or not such risk factors continue to remain operative in the development of CHD in older persons. This constitutes the third and final perspective of interactions alluded to earlier, associations between specific risk factors and CHD in older persons which will be discussed below.

Table 3 Percentage prevalence of cardiovascular risk factors in the elderly. The Framingham Study, Biennial Exam 16

Cardiovascular risk factor	*Age* (years)					
	65–74		*75–84*		*85–94*	
	Men	*Women*	*Men*	*Women*	*Men*	*Women*
Definite hypertension	42.1	48.9	45.5	61.1	20.7	64.8
Hypercholesterolemia	16.6	39.7	9.7	36.3	9.4	18.4
Glucose intolerance	29.5	17.5	30.9	26.0	33.3	29.0
Obesity	52.2	47.8	35.4	39.3	7.7	30.0
Cigarette smoking	21.9	23.0	13.9	8.5	9.4	3.2
ECG-LVH	5.5	4.2	6.0	7.8	10.4	13.0

Definite hypertension, BP > 160/95 mmHg; Hypercholesterolemia, serum cholesterol > 250 mg/dl; Glucose intolerance, blood glucose > 120 mg/dl, glucosuria or diabetes mellitus; Obesity, relative weight > 120 per cent; Cigarette smoking, any (Biennial Exam 15); ECG-LVH, evidence of left ventricular hypertrophy on electrocardiogram

ASSOCIATIONS BETWEEN SPECIFIC RISK FACTORS AND CHD IN THE ELDERLY

Associations for a number of specific risk factors and CHD are summarized in Table 4. Putative risk factors are listed in the column on the left. Standardized, age-adjusted (bivariate) logistic regression coefficients are categorized for younger and older subjects of the Framingham cohort and also arrayed separately for men and women. Regression coefficients are derived using a logistic regression model to mathematically relate the level of a risk factor or its categorical value to the development of CHD events. The magnitude of the coefficient and also the level of statistical significance reflect the strength of the association between the specific risk factor and CHD for the age group and sex under consideration.

A cursory inspection of the results indicates that the majority of significant associations between risk factors and CHD apparent in younger men and women remain significant in older age groups but not consistently in both sexes. Systolic blood pressure, for example, demonstrates strong risk associations for CHD in younger men and women and maintains strong associations in both older men and women. The risk association for diastolic blood pressure, in contrast, appears to lose significance in older women.

Table 4 Associations between specific risk factors and incidence of CHD. The Framingham Study, 30-year follow-up

	Bivariate standardized regression coefficients (age-adjusted)			
	Ages 35–64		*Ages 65–94*	
Risk factors	*Men*	*Women*	*Men*	*Women*
Systolic pressure	0.338***	0.418***	0.401***	0.286***
Diastolic pressure	0.321***	0.363***	0.296***	0.082
Serum cholesterol	0.322***	0.307***	0.121	0.213***
Cigarettes	0.259***	0.095	−0.017	−0.034
Blood glucose	0.043	0.206***	0.166***	0.209***
Vital capacity	−0.112*	−0.331***	−0.127	−0.253***
Relative weight	0.190***	0.264***	0.177**	0.124*

Significant at *$p < 0.05$, **$p < 0.01$, ***$p < 0.001$

Serum total cholesterol demonstrates strong risk associations for CHD in younger men and women, however, the strength of this risk association clearly weakens in older men but remains significant in older women. Cigarette smoking modelled using this methodology fails to show significant risk associations in either older men or women. Blood glucose levels, as well as other parameters reflecting impaired glucose metabolism including glucose intolerance and diabetes mellitus, show strong risk associations for CHD, in both older men and women. Vital capacity demonstrates strong negative risk associations, particularly in older women. Interestingly, significant risk associations between CHD and body weight expressed as Metropolitan Relative Weight are maintained in both older men and women. A number of these risk associations will be characterized in detail below.

Similar data for associations between specific risk factors and CHD incidence can be derived using an alternative regression methodology, the Cox proportional hazards model[18].

Blood pressure and hypertension

The relationship between blood pressure and CHD particularly in older persons represents one of the most striking risk associations in data from the Framingham Study. Risk relations between CHD incidence and blood pressure in men are shown in Figure 6. CHD incidence, expressed as age-adjusted annual rate of CHD events per 1000, appears on the ordinate. Systolic and diastolic blood pressures appear on the abscissas of the left and right panels, respectively. Two risk relations are illustrated in each panel, one for younger men aged 35–64 years, another for older men aged 65–94 years. Note that CHD risk for systolic and diastolic blood pressure rises with increasing pressure in both age groups and that the risk is even more striking in older than in younger men. These trends are interpreted as marked increases in relative risk indicating that progressively higher levels of blood pressure confer additional risk for CHD. Although these trends do not establish causality, they serve to emphasize an important role for blood

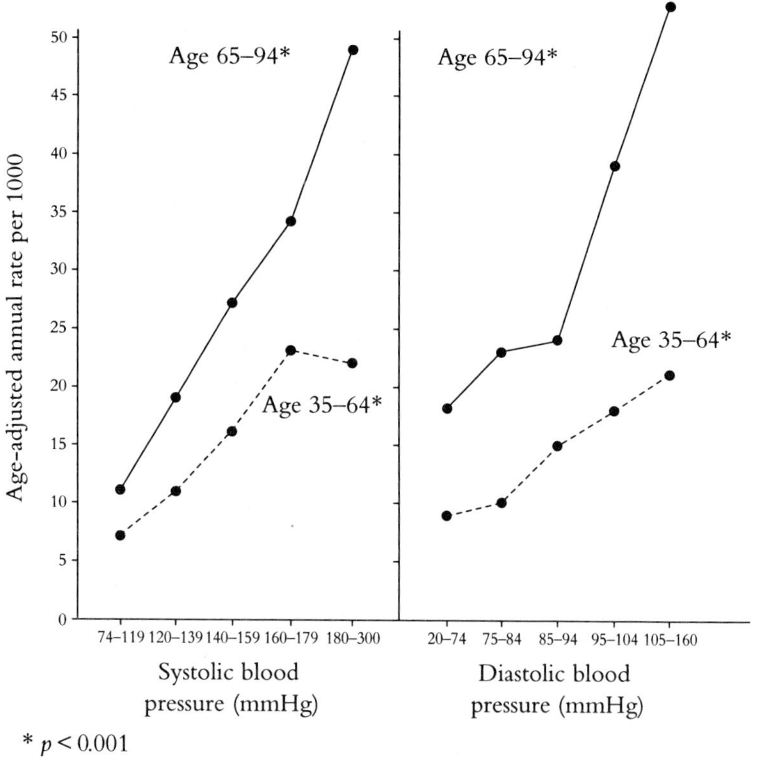

Figure 6 Risk of CHD by systolic and diastolic blood pressure according to specified age groups in men. The Framingham Study, 30-year follow-up. From reference 3, reproduced by permission

pressure in the extended sequence of pathophysiological events that result in manifest CHD. Note that risk relations in older men are configured well above those of younger men, indicating substantially higher incidence rates for CHD at similar blood pressures. This is interpreted as an increase in absolute risk for CHD in older men suggesting a substantially higher burden of disease at all levels of blood pressure in older as compared to younger men, even at normal or low blood pressures. Thus, for older men, both systolic and diastolic blood pressures confer substantial risk of similar magnitude in terms of either absolute or relative risk.

Risk relations for systolic and diastolic blood pressures in women are shown in Figure 7. Although overall incidence rates for CHD in women are lower than rates at corresponding blood pressures in men, some of the risk relations previously described in men also pertain to women. Risk appears to rise with increasing blood pressure in both age groups, i.e. increased relative risk, and incidence rates at the same level of blood pressure are higher in older than in younger women, producing an increased absolute risk. Although there is a minor deviation from the nearly linear trend for the relationship between systolic blood pressure and CHD incidence in older women, the relationship maintains strong statistical significance. In contrast, the deviation in the relationship corresponding to the fourth level of diastolic blood pressure (95–104 mmHg) yields a statistically insignificant result using the logistic regression model, despite an apparent upper curvilinear trend. Although the discontinuity in the curve remains unexplained, these findings suggest a more consistent and reliable role for systolic blood pressure as a predictor for CHD in both elderly men and women.

Risk gradients for CHD that, in general, are similar in direction and magnitude to those suggested earlier are observed when individuals are classified according to hypertensive status instead of absolute levels of blood pressure (Table 5). For all age and sex groups considered, the overall risk of CHD is two to three times higher in subjects with definite hypertension compared with normotensives, while risk is intermediate for those with mild hypertension. Absolute risk is two to three times higher in older subjects, both in men and women, and risk is nearly always higher in men than women, irrespective of age. Similar patterns of risk attributable to hypertension have been observed specifically for cerebrovascular events, congestive heart failure and peripheral vascular disease[14]. When considered alone, isolated systolic hypertension also confers substantial risk for CHD and other cardiovascular disease outcomes.

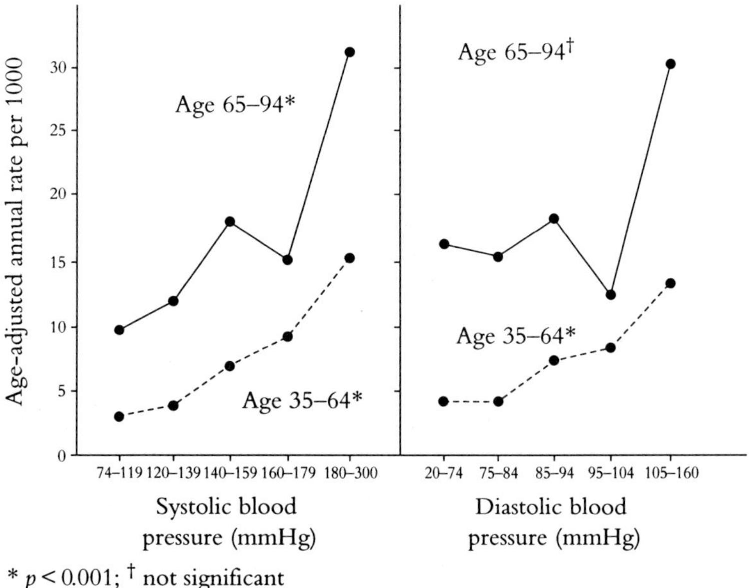

Figure 7 Risk of CHD by systolic and diastolic blood pressure according to specified age groups in women. The Framingham Study, 30-year follow-up. From reference 3, reproduced by permission

Table 5 Risk of CHD by hypertensive status according to age and sex. The Framingham Study, 30-year follow-up

	Average annual rate for CHD per 1000 (age-adjusted)			
	*Age 35–64**		*Age 65–94**	
Hypertensive status	*Men*	*Women*	*Men*	*Women*
Normal (< 140/90 mmHg)	8	3	14	11
Mild (140–160/90–95 mmHg)	15	7	28	16
Definite (> 160/95 mmHg)	21	10	41	22

*All trends significant at $p < 0.001$

Previous data from randomized clinical trials have established a strong case for the efficacy of treating combined elevations of systolic and diastolic blood pressure in older hypertensives[19,20], although considerable uncertainty remained regarding the treatment of isolated systolic hypertension. The findings of the Systolic Hypertension in the Elderly Program (SHEP) have served to dispel much of this uncertainty[21]. This study documented impressive reductions in total numbers of fatal and non-fatal strokes in the active treatment group as compared to the placebo group. Statistically significant reductions in non-fatal myocardial infarctions plus coronary death, as well as combined CHD and total cardiovascular disease outcomes, were also noted in the group on active treatment. There appeared to be little or no evidence in this study that lowering of either systolic or diastolic blood pressure resulted in an increased risk of CHD events or mortality, particularly at the lower end of the distribution for blood pressure, the so-called J-shaped curve[22].

Two other recent clinical trials of drug therapy for hypertension in the elderly that included patients with isolated systolic hypertension also showed beneficial effects[23,24]. In addition to substantial reductions in cerebrovascular events and congestive heart failure, the majority of intervention studies of drug therapy for hypertension in older persons to date have consistently demonstrated either beneficial trends or significant reductions in CHD events and mortality. Such findings appear to be considerably less prominent in clinical trials experiences derived from predominantly middle-aged hypertensives[19,20,25].

Blood lipids

The risk of CHD in older persons attributable to serum lipids represents an area of considerable uncertainty and controversy. Relations between CHD incidence and serum total cholesterol in the Framingham Study are shown in Figure 8. Separate trends are plotted in younger and older subjects for men and women, respectively. It can be seen that absolute risk is substantially increased in older as compared to younger men. Also evident is that relative risk clearly rises over the entire distribution of serum total cholesterol in younger as well as older men. The break in continuity of the risk relation at the fourth level of the distribution in older men, however, yields results that narrowly miss statistical significance both in bivariate (age-adjusted) and multivariate estimates using the logistic regression model, whereas the association remains strongly predictive in younger men. Although incidence rates for CHD at corresponding levels of cholesterol are lower in women than those in men, the same overall pattern pertains, an increase in both

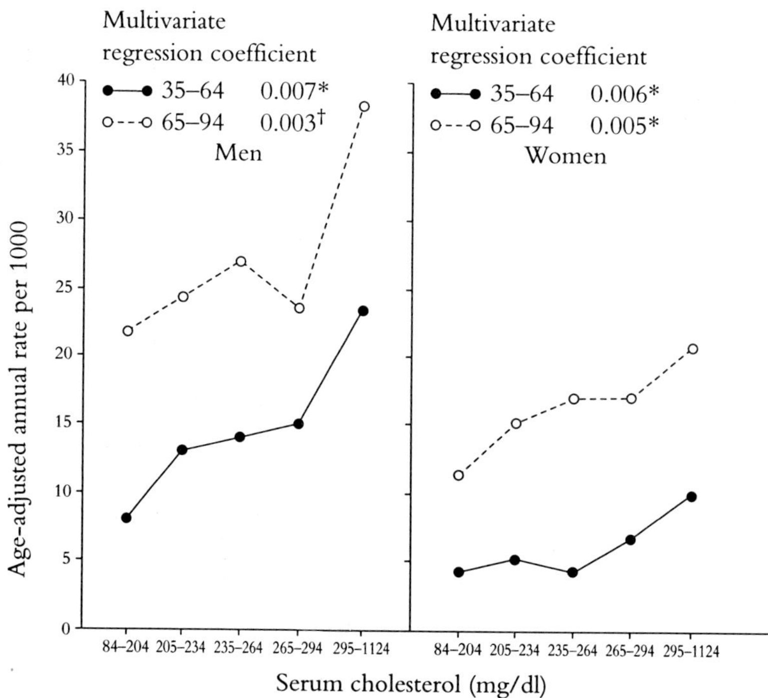

Figure 8 Risk of CHD by serum cholesterol according to specified age groups in men and women. The Framingham Study, 30-year follow-up. From reference 3, reproduced by permission
*, $p < 0.001$; †, not significant

absolute and relative risk. In this instance, however, statistical significance is maintained in both younger and older women.

The finding that serum total cholesterol loses strength as a risk factor for CHD, particularly in older men of the Framingham cohort, has resulted in serious misinterpretation by some authors who have used this information to argue that serum lipids do not represent important risk factors for CHD in the elderly and thus justify neither detection nor treatment[26,27]. This view is both extreme and unreasonable, since several other studies have clearly validated the role of serum total cholesterol as a predictor of CHD events in older men[28–34] and also older women[28,30,34]. Recent data from the Honolulu Heart Study, in particular, provide the strongest support for serum cholesterol as a potent predictor of CHD in older men[31]. Despite these findings, however, a recent meta-analysis encompassing data from 22 US and international cohort studies concluded that serum cholesterol did indeed lose strength as a risk predictor for CHD mortality in older men and also in older women[35], a finding consistent with original observations made in data from the Framingham Study. Cholesterol emerges as a significant predictor of CHD death when steps are taken to adjust for factors related to frailty or other comorbid conditions that serve to confound this risk association[36,37].

Focusing on serum cholesterol as the sole measure of risk for CHD attributable to serum lipids should now be considered obsolete, based on our current understanding of lipoprotein subfractions and the availability of standardized laboratory methods to measure them in clinical practice. Substitution of either LDL or HDL cholesterol in the regression model fully restores statistical predictability for the risk relationship between serum lipids and CHD[38]. HDL cholesterol, in particular, has emerged as an important lipid moiety that adds substantial precision in assessing coronary risk at limited additional cost[39]. Construction of a serum cholesterol/HDL ratio provides a highly accurate characterization of CHD risk in older men and women in the Framingham Study, which is illustrated in Figure 9. Indeed, data from Framingham as well as other studies confirm the overall reliability of the cholesterol/HDL ratio in assessing CHD risk in younger and older persons and in men as well as women[30,38,40,41]. The rationale for this approach is that the ratio reliably captures the effect of a dynamic equilibrium of lipid transport into and out of body tissues possibly including the intima of blood vessels.

Several studies have suggested that serum triglycerides may be important predictors for CHD in either older men or older women, but not consistently in both sexes[30,38,40,42]. Despite these observations, the present consensus holds that elevated levels of serum triglycerides represent a risk marker for obesity, glucose intolerance and low HDL levels, all of which confer risk for CHD and as such deserve preventive attention.

Data from intervention studies using dietary measures or drug therapy demonstrate the benefit of lipid alteration in reducing the risk of CHD events particularly in middle-aged men[43,44]. Systematic information from clinical trials regarding the efficacy and safety of treating lipid abnormalities in the elderly, despite their prevalence in this population, is not yet available. A strong case for the widespread application of drug therapy to reduce risk of CHD in older persons as an element of primary prevention is not warranted at the present time. Of considerable interest is the information from two large clinical trials, which makes a compelling case for reducing

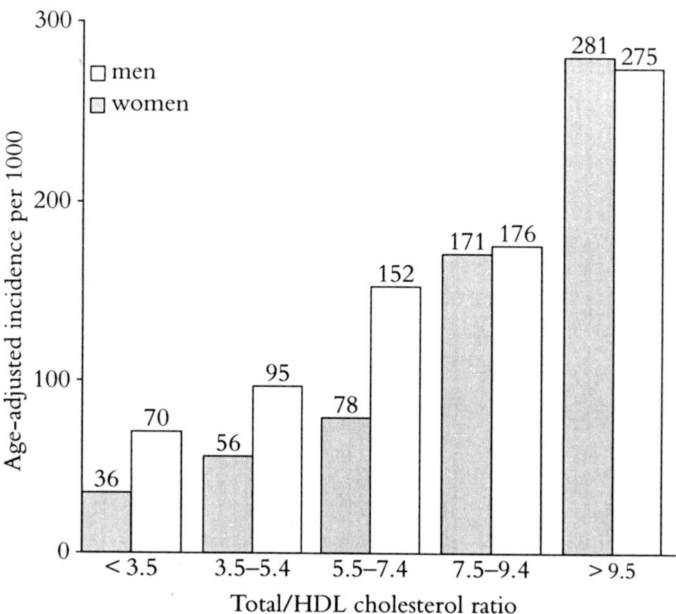

Figure 9   Risk of CHD by total/HDL cholesterol ratios among men and women aged 50–90 years. The Framingham Study, 26-year follow-up

elevated or even average levels of LDL cholesterol with drugs in patients with established CHD, angina pectoris or following myocardial infarction[45,46]. These effects of drug therapy in the secondary prevention of CHD events, in persons with pre-existing CHD, appear to be beneficial in both middle-aged and older patients of both sexes.

Current management of hypercholesterolemia for an older person considered to be at risk, should consist of a highly individualized approach beginning with appropriate dietary measures and weight control before initiating a trial of specific drug therapy, preferably at lower doses, to achieve a carefully monitored lipid-lowering effect[47].

Cigarette smoking

Cigarette smoking fails to demonstrate strong risk associations for total CHD events in either older men or older women using the logistic regression methodology indicated in Table 4. Significant risk associations, however, are discerned between cigarette smoking and death due to CHD[9]. One interpretation of this phenomenon is that smoking may be more closely related to lethal events alone than to outcomes comprised of combinations of morbid and lethal events[48]. A more likely explanation is that the cross-sectional pooling approach used in the analysis may classify long-term smokers who have discontinued cigarettes for relatively brief periods as non-smokers, in effect diluting the strength of the association between the risk factor and the outcome[49]. Because of these difficulties, the most reliable approach in assessing risk associations between cigarette smoking and cardiovascular morbidity or mortality is to model these events prospectively for defined categories of smoking behaviors (e.g. current smoker, former smoker and never smoker) and for longer time intervals. Such approaches yield strong risk associations between cigarette smoking and a broad array of cardiovascular outcomes including CHD, stroke and peripheral arterial disease, even in older men and women. These observations have been documented using data from Framingham as well as other studies[30,50–52].

Reducing the risk of cardiovascular disease is not the only reason to encourage discontinuation of cigarettes in older persons. Cigarettes contribute to the development of chronic bronchitis and obstructive lung disease as well as lung cancer and other malignancies. These conditions also exact a heavy toll in terms of disability and death in the elderly. Thus, the clinician can make a compelling case that it is never too late to stop smoking and extend appropriate advice and encouragement to assist patients in their effort to discontinue cigarettes.

Glucose tolerance and diabetes mellitus

Impaired glucose metabolism is not only highly prevalent in the elderly but also confers substantial risk for CHD as well as other cardiovascular events in both older men and women. Various measures of glucose tolerance are employed and nearly all demonstrate significant risk associations with CHD in the Framingham Study[9]. These measures include blood glucose levels, glycosuria and the composite risk categories designated as glucose intolerance and diabetes mellitus. Although diabetes mellitus confers enhanced risk for both younger and older men, overall risk increases dramatically for both younger and older women[53] (Figure 10). Similar patterns of risk are noted for coronary and cardiovascular mortality[9,53]. Diabetes also emerges as an important risk factor in the development of congestive heart failure,

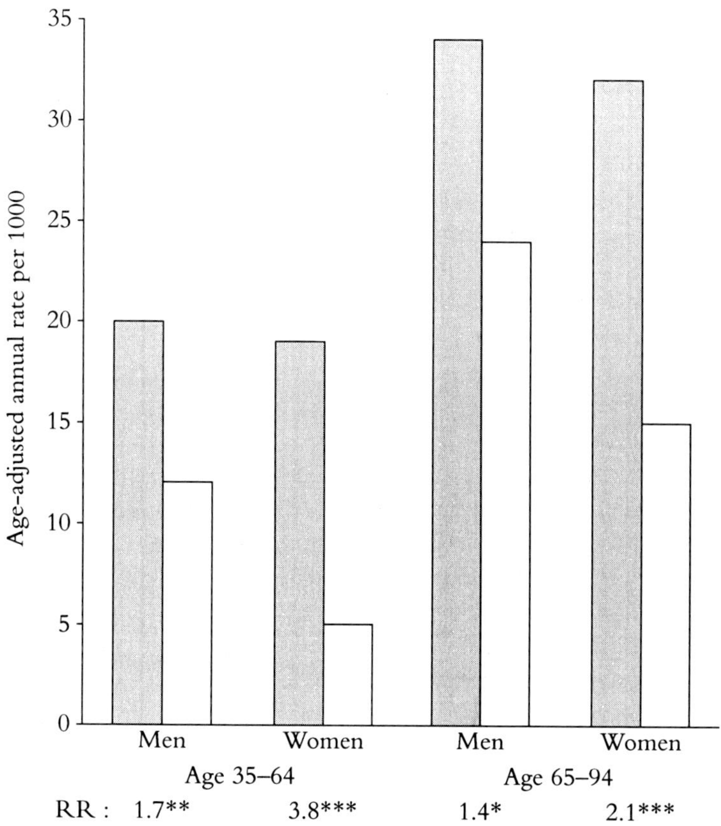

Figure 10 Age-adjusted incidence rates for CHD based on diabetic status classified according to age and sex. Solid bar, diabetic; open bar, non-diabetic; RR, risk ratio diabetic/non-diabetic. From reference 53, reproduced by permission ***, $p < 0.001$; **, $p < 0.01$; *, $p < 0.05$

particularly in older women with insulin-dependent diabetes mellitus[54]. Presumably, the microvascular disease that is unique to diabetes, combined with other mechanisms, serves to produce progressive damage to heart muscle, ultimately resulting in compromised ventricular function and heart failure.

There is little evidence that control of hyperglycemia, either by oral hypoglycemic agents or insulin, effectively forestalls either complications or the development of cardiovascular disease[53,55] although encouraging trends in this regard were identified in the recently completed Diabetes Control and Complications Trial[56]. Available evidence would, therefore, suggest that there is more to be gained in reducing risk by correcting associated cardiovascular risk factors in persons with diabetes than by attention confined to early detection and control of hyperglycemia.

Left ventricular hypertrophy

Left ventricular hypertrophy as determined by the electrocardiogram (ECG-LVH) emerges as a strong risk factor for CHD in older men and women (Figure 11). Marked increases in CHD incidence are noted for voltage criteria for LVH alone, with additional risk conferred by definite LVH which, in addition to voltage criteria, includes repolarization (ST and T wave) abnormalities consistent with LVH. These electrocardiographic findings presumably reflect abnormalities of myocardial structure and function related to early compromise of the underlying coronary circulation that antedate the development of clinical manifestations of CHD[57–59].

In this context, left ventricular hypertrophy (LV mass) as determined by echocardiography has emerged as an extremely potent independent predictor of CHD and other cardiovascular disease events especially in older persons[60,61].

Body weight

Of considerable interest is the discovery that increased body weight represents a significant risk marker for CHD even at advanced age. The association between body weight and risk for CHD in older subjects of the Framingham Study is illustrated in Figure 12. It is notable that while CHD risk rises more strikingly with increasing body weight in older men, trends in older women clearly indicate enhanced risk at higher body weights. Progressive increases in body weight occurring earlier in life correlate closely with changes in the levels of several risk factors considered to be more directly related to pathogenesis of atherosclerosis[62]. These include increases in blood pressure, serum cholesterol, triglycerides and blood glucose with a reduction in HDL cholesterol. These findings serve to emphasize the need to incorporate measures ultimately designed to either control or, if necessary, to gradually reduce body weight as part of risk management even in

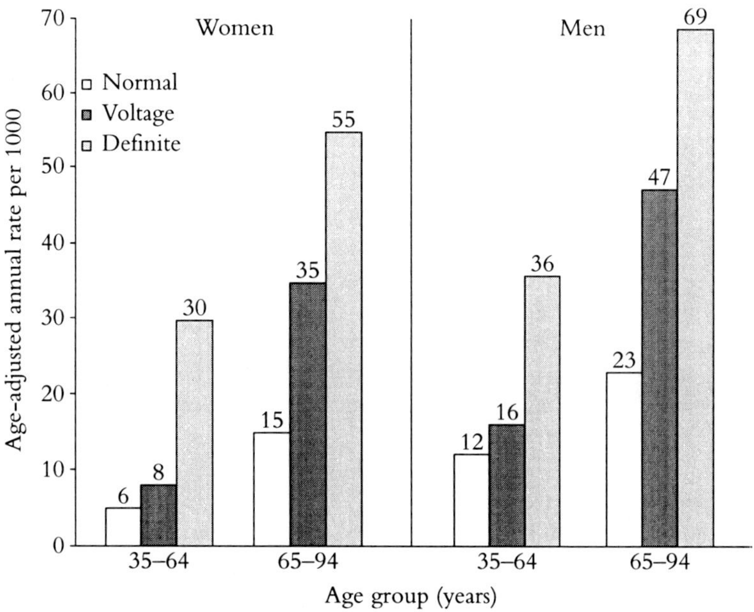

Figure 11 Risk of CHD according to ECG-LVH status. The Framingham Study, 30-year follow-up

older persons. When coupled with appropriate dietary measures, weight control would be particularly useful in the initial management of elderly patients with hypertension, dyslipidemia and diabetes or combinations of these conditions.

Physical activity

Accumulating evidence now suggests that vigorous physical activity during the lifetime may forestall CHD in the elderly[63–65]. Previously reported data from Framingham indicated that overall mortality, including coronary mortality, was inversely related to the level of physical activity in middle-aged men[66]. A benefit for exercise in older men was also suggested, although the levels of exercise involved were quite modest. Although regular physical

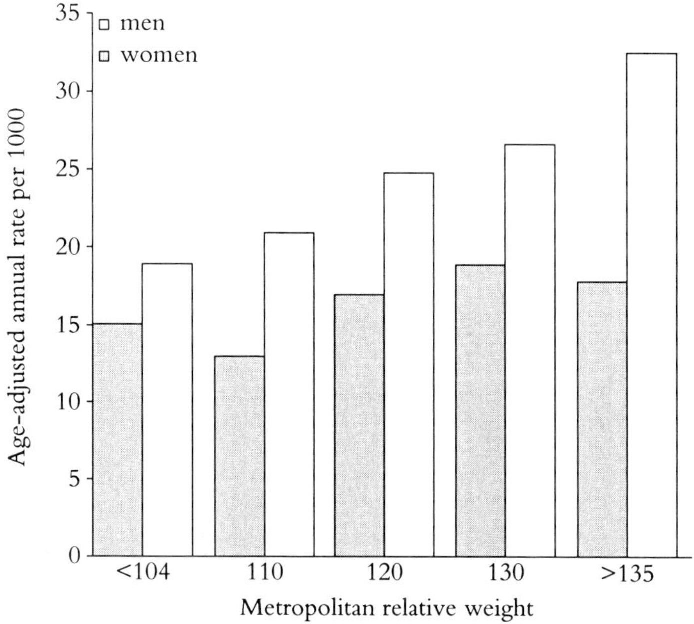

Figure 12 Risk of CHD according to body weight in men and women, aged 65–94 years. The Framingham Study, 30-year follow-up

activity in the elderly is desirable and should be strongly encouraged, it would be unwise to place undue emphasis on this approach alone in attempting to reduce the risk for CHD.

Prevalent CHD

An important predictor of CHD events at all ages is the presence of antecedent CHD. It is therefore of interest that several of the risk factors associated with the initial development of CHD in the elderly not only continue to have strong correlations with prevalent disease, but also maintain predictive associations for new CHD events in older persons with pre-existing disease[30,32,67–69]. Serum lipids, cigarette smoking and diabetes appear to be more prominent in this context than hypertension. Blood pressure may fall substantially following myocardial infarction, particularly extensive anterior myocardial infarction which carries a poorer prognosis, thereby confounding the relationship between hypertension and CHD morbidity and mortality[70]. Blood pressure, however, re-emerges as a significant predictor of recurrent CHD events in long-term survivors of myocardial infarction[71].

These findings serve to emphasize the critical role of controlling risk factors in older persons with established CHD. Effective treatment of hypertension, discontinuation of cigarettes and adequate control of hyperglycemia are important measures in the preventive clinical management of such individuals. The potential benefit of lipid-lowing drugs in older persons with established CHD and hypercholesterolemia was alluded to earlier.

Other risk factors

Several hematological or hemostatic factors have been described as risk variables in the Framingham Study. Hematocrit appeared to contribute to CHD in younger men and women in this analysis, but not in older persons[9]. White blood cell count, which was strongly correlated with the number of cigarettes smoked per day, hematocrit and vital capacity, was also associated with enhanced risk for CHD and other cardiovascular end-points in older men, both in smokers and non-smokers, but only in those women who smoked[72]. These data were consistent with reports from other studies[73]. Plasma fibrinogen showed strong risk associations for CHD and other cardiovascular disease outcomes in men including older men[74] similar to findings from other studies[75]. Significant risk associations, however, were not apparent in older women.

An extensive array of psychosocial, occupational, dietary and other factors have been described as putative risk parameters for CHD in the Framingham Study[76], however, only limited information is available regarding specific associations of these factors with CHD in older persons. Although family history of CHD is strongly related to early development of CHD (before the age of 60) in both men and women in the Framingham Study, predictive associations also remained significant for the late onset of CHD[77].

CHD RISK PROFILES IN THE ELDERLY

Although associations between a specific risk factor and CHD can be considered in isolation as a single relationship, in many instances combinations of several risk factors may constitute the observed risk profile, especially in older persons. Risk of CHD, in such instances, can be reliably estimated by synthesizing a number of risk factors into a composite score, based on a multiple logistic function[78]. Risk factors are assessed by standard clinical procedures (smoking history, blood pressure and electrocardiogram) and by routine laboratory studies (serum total cholesterol, HDL cholesterol and blood glucose). This type of composite index permits detection of individuals at relatively high risk, either on the basis of marked elevation of a single factor or because of marginal abnormalities of several risk factors.

This multivariate risk scenario is illustrated in Figure 13 which characterizes the risk of CHD at two predefined levels of serum cholesterol and then considers changes in the levels or values of other risk factors towards worsening risk, as indicated in the lower part of the figure below. Note that risk increases progressively with the additional impact of other risk factors for both categories of serum cholesterol, even in instances where a factor such as cigarette smoking has a relatively weak risk association with CHD when considered alone.

The major risk factors including age, when taken together, explain only a limited proportion of the variance of CHD incidence in younger as well

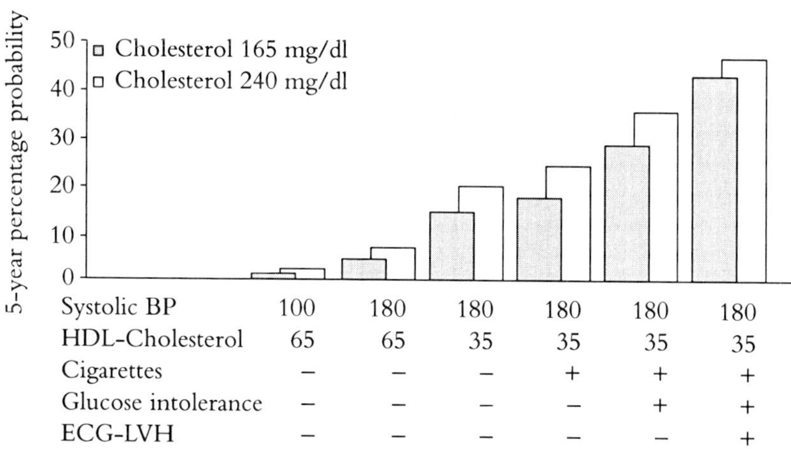

Systolic BP	100	180	180	180	180	180
HDL-Cholesterol	65	65	35	35	35	35
Cigarettes	–	–	–	+	+	+
Glucose intolerance	–	–	–	–	+	+
ECG-LVH	–	–	–	–	–	+

Figure 13 Risk of CHD of two levels of serum cholesterol according to specified levels or categories of other risk factors for 70-year-old women in the Framingham Study

as older persons[78]. It is likely that other major risk attributes exist among both the young and the elderly, but are yet to be identified. It must be emphasized, however, that the factors that have already been delineated do identify high-risk subgroups of the elderly population that should be targeted for preventive management.

PERSPECTIVES FOR PRIMARY PREVENTION OF CHD IN THE ELDERLY

An important principle of prevention is the concept that measures limiting the effect of known risk factors should be initiated as early in life as possible to minimize the subsequent development of disease in both the young and the elderly. It is unreasonable to conclude, however, that modifications of risk factors initiated at advanced age are likely to be ineffective in reducing the toll of related disease in older persons. A simple but important observation in this context is that the incidence of CHD in the elderly varies widely within distributions of continuous risk factors such as blood pressure or serum cholesterol. Incidence also appears to differ markedly for values of categorical variables such as the presence or absence of left ventricular hypertrophy. In addition, data presented earlier indicate that the incidence of CHD, as well as other cardiovascular disease events, is not only substantially higher in populations of older persons but also continues to rise with advancing age across the life span. Because incidence is usually higher in older persons, the beneficial effect of a given intervention such as treatment of hypertension or hypercholesterolemia, as assessed by reduction in relative risk, may be similar to or lower than that observed in younger persons[2,3,19,47,79]. In many such instances, however, the same effect measured as a difference in absolute risk, reflecting reduction in numerical toll of disease outcomes, actually remains higher in the elderly. A corollary of this effect is that a smaller number of older as compared to younger people must be treated to yield the same benefit in terms of numbers of disease events prevented. These considerations are more relevant today than ever before.

Recently, a marked and progressive decline in mortality due to coronary and cardiovascular disease has occurred in the United States and several other industrialized nations[80]. Age-specific trends indicate decreasing mortality due to CHD and cardiovascular disease, both in the elderly and in younger adults of both sexes. Similar trends in cardiovascular mortality have been identified in the Framingham population[81]. At the same time, the prevalence of several coronary risk factors, such as untreated hypertension, elevated serum cholesterol levels and cigarette smoking, has diminished in the population at large, including the elderly, while impressive improvements have occurred in the diagnosis and treatment of CHD. Although the available information supports the contention that both of these potentially beneficial effects have contributed to the observed decline in mortality from CHD, the present consensus gives greater weight to the success of widespread primary preventive strategies, resulting in lowered levels of major risk factors that contribute to disease, rather than to improved diagnosis and treatment of established disease[82].

In this context, hypertension clearly emerges as the dominant, potentially remediable, risk factor for both CHD and cerebrovascular disease morbidity and mortality in the elderly. Hypertension is highly prevalent in the aged, easily detected, and can be corrected by the careful application of appropriate measures, including drug therapy. As mentioned earlier, direct evidence from clinical trials has already established the efficacy of antihypertensive measures in reducing the frequency of both stroke and CHD events in elderly hypertensives. Available information also makes a compelling case for discontinuation of cigarettes at all ages, including the elderly. Information is needed, however, regarding the feasibility and effectiveness of non-pharmacological approaches such as diet and weight reduction in treating older persons with hypertension and lipid abnormalities both as initial therapy and as adjuncts to specific drug therapy. Also, as a matter of critical importance, the efficacy and safety of drug therapy for the treatment of lipid abnormalities in the elderly for the purpose of primary prevention should be established in large, well-designed clinical trials. Lack of such information severely limits our confidence in extending what may be a potentially beneficial preventive measure to greater numbers of older persons.

ACKNOWLEDGEMENTS

The authors wish to thank Ms Claire Chisholm for her invaluable assistance in preparing this manuscript. This work was supported by the Health Services Research and Development Service of the Department of Veterans

Affairs, the Visiting Scientist Program of the Framingham Heart Study and grant nos. NO1-HV-92922, NO1-HV52971 and 5T32-HL-07374-13 of the National Institutes of Health.

REFERENCES

1. Kannel, W. B. and Gordon T. (1978) Evaluation of cardiovascular risk in the elderly: the Framingham Study. *Bull. NY Acad. Med.*, **54**, 573–91

2. Kannel, W. B. and Vokonas, P. S. (1986). Primary risk factors for coronary heart disease in the elderly: the Framingham study. In Wenger, N. K., Furberg, C. D., Pitt, E. eds. *Coronary Heart Disease in the Elderly*. New York: Elsevier Science Publishing, 60–92

3. Vokonas, P. S. and Kannel, W. B. (1993). Epidemiology of coronary heart disease in the elderly. In Tresch, D. D. and Aronow, W. S. eds. *Cardiovascular Disease in the Elderly Patient*. New York: Marcel Dekker, Inc., 91–123

4. Kannel, W. B. and Vokonas, P. S. (1992). Demographics of prevalence, incidence and management of coronary heart disease in the elderly and in women. *Ann. Epidemiol.*, **2**, 5–14

5. Rich, M. (1990). Acute myocardial infarction in the elderly. *Cardiology*, **7**, 79–90

6. Forman, D. E., Bernal, J. L. G. and Wei, J. Y. (1992). Management of acute myocardial infarction in the very elderly. *Am. J. Med.*, **93**, 315–26

7. Wenger, N. K. (1992). Cardiovascular disease in the elderly. *Curr. Probl. Cardiol.*, **10**, 615–90

8. Lakatta, E. G. (1985). Cardiovascular function in later life. *Cardiovasc. Med.*, **10**, 37–40

9. Cupples, L. A. and D'Agostino, R. B. (1987). Section 34. Some risk factors related to the annual incidence of cardiovascular disease and death using pooled repeated biennial measurements: Framingham Heart Study, 30-year follow-up. In: Kannel, W. B., Wolf, P. A., Garrison, R. J. eds. *The Framingham Study: An Epidemiological Investigation of Cardiovascular Disease*. Bethesda, MD, National Heart, Lung, and Blood Institute publication No. (NIH) 87-2703

10. Kannel, W. B. and Abbott, R. D. (1984). Incidence and prognosis of unrecognized myocardial infarction: an update from the Framingham Study. *N. Engl. J. Med.*, **11**, 1144–7

11. Learoyd, B. M. and Taylor, M. G. (1966). Alterations with age in the viscoelastic properties of human arterial walls. *Circ. Res.*, **18**, 278–92

12. Maddocks, I. (1976). Possible absence of essential hypertension in two complete Pacific Island populations. *Lancet*, **2**, 327–31

13. Avolio, A. P., Deng, F. Q., Li, W. G. *et al.* (1985). Effects of aging on arterial distensibility in populations with high and low prevalence of hypertension: comparison between urban and rural communities in China. *Circulation*, **71**, 202–10

14. Vokonas, P. S., Kannel, W. B. and Cupples, L. A. (1988). Epidemiology and risk of hypertension in the elderly: the Framingham Study. *J. Hypertens.*, **8** (Suppl. 1) 53–9

15. Wilking, S. V., Belanger, A. J., Kannel, W. B. *et al.* (1988). Determinants of isolated systolic hypertension. *J. Am. Med. Assoc.*, **260**, 3451–5

16. DeFronzo, R. A. (1981). Glucose intolerance and aging. *Diabetes Care*, **4**, 493–501

17. Borkan, G. A. and Norris, A. H. (1977). Fat redistribution and the changing body dimensions of the adult male. *Human Biology*, **49**, 495–514

18. Harris, T., Cook, E. F., Kannel, W. B. *et al.* (1988). Proportional hazards analysis of risk factors for coronary heart disease in individuals 65 or older. The Framingham Heart Study. *J. Am. Geriatric Soc.*, **36**, 1023–8

19. Applegate, W. B. (1989). Hypertension in elderly patients. *Ann. Intern. Med.*, **110**, 901–15

20. Mulrow, C. D., Cornell, J. A., Herrero, C. R. *et al.* (1994). Hypertension in the elderly: implications and generalizability of randomized trials. *J. Am. Med. Assoc.*, **272**, 1932–8

21. SHEP Cooperative Research Group. (1991). Prevention of stroke by anti-hypertensive drug treatment in older persons with isolated systolic hypertension: final results of the Systolic Hypertension in the Elderly Program (SHEP). *J. Am. Med. Assoc.*, **265**, 3255–64

22. Cruickshank, J. M., Thorp, J. M. and Zacharias, F. J. (1987). Benefits and potential harm of lowering high blood pressure. *Lancet*, **1**, 581–4

23. Dahlof, B., Lindholm, L. H., Hausson, L. *et al.* (1991). Morbidity and mortality in the Swedish Trial in Old Patients with Hypertension (STOP-Hypertension). *Lancet*, **338**, 1281–5

24. MRC Working Party. (1992). Medical Research Council trial of treatment of hypertension in older adults: principal results. *Br. Med. J.*, **304**, 405–12

25. Strandgaard, S. and Haunso, S. (1987). Why does anti-hypertensive treatment prevent stroke but not myocardial infarction? *Lancet*, **2**, 658–61

26. Hulley, S. B. and Newman, T. B. (1994). Cholesterol in the elderly. Is it important? (Editorial) *J. Am. Med. Assoc.*, **272**, 1372–4

27. Garber, A. M., Browner, W. S., Mazzaferri, E. L. *et al.* (1996). Guidelines for using serum cholesterol, high density lipoprotein cholesterol, and triglyceride levels as screening tests for preventing coronary heart disease in adults. *Ann. Intern. Med.*, **124**, 515–17

28. Barret-Connor, E., Suarez, L., Khaw, K. T. *et al.* (1984). Ischemic heart disease factors after age 50. *J. Chronic Diseases*, **37**, 903–8

29. Stamler, J., Wentworth, D. and Neaton, J. D. (1986) for the MRFIT Research Group. Is the relationship between serum cholesterol and risk of premature death from coronary heart disease continuous and graded? Findings in 356,222 primary screenees of the Multiple Risk Factor Intervention Trial (MRFIT). *J. Am. Med. Assoc.*, **256**, 2835–8

30. Aronow, W. S., Herzig, A. H., Etienne, F. *et al.* (1989). 41-month follow-up of risk factors correlated with new coronary events in 708 elderly patients. *J. Am. Geriatric Soc.*, **37**, 501–6

31. Benfante, R. and Reed, D. (1990). Is elevated serum cholesterol level a factor for coronary heart disease in the elderly? *J. Am. Med. Assoc.*, **263**, 393–6

32. Pikkanen, J., Linn, S., Heiss, G. *et al.* (1990). Ten-year mortality from cardiovascular disease in relation to cholesterol level among men with and without preexisting cardiovascular disease. *N. Engl. J. Med.*, **322**, 1700–7

33. Sorkin, J. D., Andres, R., Muller, D. C. *et al.* (1992). Cholesterol as a risk factor for coronary heart disease in elderly men. The Baltimore Longitudinal Study of Aging. *Ann. Epidemiol.*, **2**, 59–67

34. Keil, J. E., Sutherland, S. E., Knapp, R. G. *et al.* (1992). Serum cholesterol – risk factor for coronary heart disease mortality in younger and older blacks and whites. The Charleston Heart Study, 1960–1988. *Ann. Epidemiol.*, **2**, 93–9

35. Manolio, T. A., Pearson, T. A., Wenger, N. K. *et al.* (1992). Cholesterol and heart disease in older persons and women: review of an NHLBI Workshop. *Ann. Epidemiol.*, **2**, 161–76

36. Corti, M. C., Guralnik, J. M. and Salive, M. E. (1997). Clarifying the direct relation between total cholesterol levels and death from coronary heart disease in older persons. *Ann. Intern. Med.*, **126**, 753–9

37. Jacobs, D., Blackburn, H., Higgins, H. M. *et al.* (1992). Report of the Conference on Low Blood Cholesterol: mortality associations. *Circulation*, **86**, 1045–60

38. Castelli, W. P., Wilson, P. W. F., Levy, D. *et al.* (1989). Cardiovascular risk factors in the elderly. *Am. J. Cardiol.*, **63**, 12H–19H

39. Corti, M. C., Guralnik, J. M., Salive, M. E. *et al.* (1995). HDL cholesterol predicts coronary heart disease mortality in older adults. *J. Am. Med. Assoc.*, **274**, 539–44

40. Castelli, W. P., Anderson, K., Wilson, P. W. F. *et al.* (1992). Lipids and risk of coronary heart disease. The Framingham Study. *Ann. Epidemiol.*, **2**, 23–8

41. Hong, M. K., Romm, P. A., Reagan, K. *et al.* (1991). Total cholesterol/HDL ratio is the best predictor of anatomic coronary artery disease among elderly patients (Abstract). *J. Am. Coll. Cardiol.*, **17**, 151A

42. Gotto, A. M. Jr. (1992). Hypertriglyceridemia: risks and perspectives. *Am. J. Cardiol.*, **70**, 19H–25H

43. Levine, G. N., Keaney, J. F. Jr and Vita, J. A. (1995). Cholesterol reduction in cardiovascular disease: clinical benefits and possible mechanisms. *N. Eng. J. Med.*, **332**, 512–19

44. Shepherd, J., Cobbe, S. M., Ford, I. *et al.* for the West of Scotland Coronary Prevention Study Group. (1995). Prevention of coronary heart disease with pravastatin in men with hypercholesterolemia. *N. Eng. J. Med.*, **333**, 1301–7

45. Scandinavian Simvastatin Survival Study Group. (1994). Randomized trial of cholesterol lowering in 4444 patients with coronary heart disease. The Scandinavian Simvastatin Survival Study (4S). *Lancet*, **344**, 1383–9

46. Sacks, F. M., Pfeffer, M. A., Moye, L. A. *et al.* for the Cholesterol and Recurrent Events Trial Investigators. (1996). The effects of pravastatin on coronary events after myocardial infarction in patients with average cholesterol levels. *N. Engl. J. Med.*, **335**, 1001–9

47. Denke, M. A. and Grundy, S. M. (1990). Hypercholesterolemia in elderly persons: resolving the treatment dilemma. *Ann. Intern. Med.*, **112**, 780–92

48. Muller, J. E., Abela, G. S., Nesto, R. W. *et al.* (1994). Triggers, acute risk factors and vulnerable plaques: the lexicon of a new frontier. *J. Am. Coll. Cardiol.*, **23**, 809–13

49. Cupples, L. A., D'Agostino, R. B., Anderson, K. *et al.* (1988). Comparison of baseline and repeated measure covariate techniques in the Framingham Heart Study. *Stat. In Med.*, **7**, 205–18

50. Kannel, W. B. and Higgins, M. (1990). Smoking and hypertension as predictors of cardiovascular risk in population studies. *J. Hypertens.*, **8** (Suppl. 5), S3–S8

51. Benfante, R., Reed, D. and Frank, J. (1991). Does smoking have an independent effect on coronary heart disease incidence in the elderly? *Am. J. Public Health*, **81**, 897–9

52. LaCroix, A. Z., Lang, J., Scherr, P. *et al.* (1991). Smoking and mortality among older men and women in three communities. *N. Engl. J. Med.*, **324**, 1619–25

53. Vokonas, P. S. and Kannel, W. B. (1996). Diabetes mellitus and coronary heart disease in the elderly. In Aronow, W. and Tresch, D. (eds.) *Clinics in Geriatric Medicine*. Philadelphia: W. B. Saunders Co. **12(1)**, 69–78

54. Kannel, W. B., Hjortland, M. and Castelli, W. B. (1970). Role of diabetes in congestive heart failure: the Framingham Study. *Ann. Intern. Med.*, **72**, 813–22

55. Wilson, P. W. F., Cupples, L. and Kannel, W. B. (1991). Is hyperglycemia associated with cardiovascular disease? The Framingham Study. *Am. Heart J.*, **121**, 586–90

56. Diabetes Control and Complications Trial Research Group (1993). The effect of intensive treatment of diabetes in the development and progression of long-term complications in insulin-dependent diabetes mellitus. *N. Engl. J. Med.*, **329**, 977–86

57. Kannel, W. B., Dannenberg, A. L. and Levy, D. (1987). Population implications of electrocardiographic left ventricular hypertrophy. *Am. J. Cardiol.*, **60**, 851–931

58. Aronow, W. S. (1992). Left ventricular hypertrophy. *J. Am. Geriatr. Soc.*, **40**, 71–80

59. Levy, D., Salomon, M. and D'Agostino, R. B. (1994). Prognostic implications of baseline electrocardiographic features and their serial changes in subjects with left-ventricular hypertrophy. *Circulation.*, **90**, 1786–93

60. Aronow, W. S., Koenigsberg, M. and Schwartz, K. S. (1988). Usefulness of echocardiographic left ventricular hypertrophy in predicting new coronary events and atherothrombotic brain infarction in patients over 62 years of age. *Am. J. Cardiol.*, **61**, 1130–2

61. Levy, D., Garrison, R. J., Savage, D. D. *et al.* (1989). Left ventricular mass and incidence of coronary disease in an elderly cohort. The Framingham Heart Study. *Ann. Intern. Med.*, **110**, 101–7

62. Borkan, G. A., Sparrow, D., Wisnieski, C. *et al.* (1986). Body weight and coronary risk: patterns of risk factor change associated with long-term weight change. The Normative Aging Study. *Am. J. Epidemiol.*, **124(3)**, 410–19

63. Donahue, R. P., Abbott, R. D., Reed, D. M. *et al.* (1988). Physical activity and coronary heart disease in middle-aged and elderly men: the Honolulu Heart Program. *Am. J. Public Health*, **78**, 683–5

64. Berlin, J. A. and Colditz, G. A. (1990). A meta-analysis of physical activity in the prevention of coronary heart disease. *Am. J. Epidemiol.*, **132**, 612–28

65. Paffenbarger, R. S. Jr, Hyde, R. T., Wing, A. L. *et al.* (1993). The association of changes in physical activity level and other lifestyle characteristics with mortality among men. *N. Engl. J. Med.*, **328**, 533–7

66. Kannel, W. B., Belanger, A. J., D'Agostino, R. B. *et al.* (1986). Physical activity and physical demand on the job and risk of cardiovascular disease and death: the Framingham Study. *Am. Heart J.*, **112**, 820–5

67. Wong, N. D., Wilson, P. W. F. and Kannel, W. B. (1991). Serum cholesterol as a prognostic factor after myocardial infarction. The Framingham Study. *Ann. Intern. Med.*, **115**, 687–97

68. Simons, L. A., Friedlander, Y., McCallum, J. *et al.* (1991). The Dubbo Study of health of the elderly: correlates of coronary heart disease at study entry. *J. Am. Geriatric Soc.*, **39**, 584–90

69. Applegate, W. B., Hughes, J. P. and Vander-Zwaag, R. (1991). Case-control study of coronary heart disease risk factors in the elderly. *J. Clin. Epidemiol.*, **44**, 409–15

70. Kannel, W. B., Sorlie, P. D., Castelli, W. P. *et al.* (1980). Blood pressure and survival after myocardial infarction. The Framingham Study. *Am. J. Cardiol.*, **45**, 326–30

71. Wong, N. D., Cupples, L. A., Ostfeld, A. M. *et al.* (1989). Risk factors for long-term coronary prognosis after initial myocardial infarction. The Framingham Study. *Am. J. Epidemiol.*, **130**, 469–80

72. Kannel, W. B., Anderson, K. and Wilson, P. W. F. (1992). White blood cell count and cardiovascular disease. *J. Am. Med. Assoc.*, **267**, 1253–6

73. de Labry, L. O., Campion, E. W., Glynn, R. J. *et al.* (1990). White blood cell count as a long term predictor of mortality: results over 18 years from the Normative Aging Study. *J. Clin. Epidemiol.*, **43**, 153–7

74. Kannel, W. B., Wolf, P. A., Castelli, W. P. *et al.* (1987). Fibrinogen and risk of cardiovascular disease. The Framingham Study. *J. Am. Med. Assoc.*, **258**, 1183–6

75. Ernst, E. (1994). Fibrinogen: its emerging role as a cardiovascular risk factor. *Angiology*, **45**, 87–93

76. Kannel, W. B. and Eaker, E. D. (1986). Psychosocial and other features of coronary heart disease: insights from the Framingham Study. *Am. Heart J.*, **112**, 1066–73

77. Schildkraut, J. M., Myers, R. H., Cupples, L. A. *et al.* (1989). Coronary risk associated with age and sex of parental heart disease in the Framingham Study. *Am. J. Cardiol.*, **64**, 555–9

78. Chambless, L. E., Dobson, A. J., Patterson, C. C. *et al.* (1990). On the use of logistic risk score in predicting risk of coronary heart disease. *Stat. Med.*, **9**, 385–96

79. Malenka, D. J. and Baron, J. A. (1988). Cholesterol and coronary heart disease. The importance of patient-specific attributable risk. *Arch. Intern. Med.*, **148**, 2247–52

80. Walker, W. J. (1983). Changing U.S. life style and declining vascular mortality – a retrospective. *N. Engl. J. Med.*, **308**, 649–51

81. Sytkowski, P. A., Kannel, W. B. and D'Agostino, R. B. (1990). Changes in risk factors and the decline in mortality from cardiovascular disease. The Framingham Heart Study. *N. Engl. J. Med.*, **322**, 1635–41

82. Goldman, L. (1990). Cost-effectiveness perspectives in coronary heart disease. *Am. Heart J.*, **119**, 733–9

2

Prediction and prevention of coronary disease in the elderly

L. A. Simons

INTRODUCTION

The prevention of coronary artery disease (CAD) in any age group depends, in part, on how reliably one can predict the disease with causal or risk factors – the observational studies. Secondly, prevention also depends on the demonstration of successful outcomes in controlled, clinical trials – the interventional studies. This paper will address current knowledge in relation to observational studies and will add new findings currently being generated in the Australian elderly. The paper will also briefly place in perspective the results of interventional studies as they apply to the elderly.

OBSERVATIONAL STUDIES

The risk factors for CAD in middle-aged subjects have been well defined and consistently include hypertension, cigarette smoking, lipid disorders, diabetes and family history[1-5]. Risk-factor prediction by many of these factors in the elderly is more complex. Hypertension has been shown to be predictive of CAD in the elderly[6-8], although low blood pressure may predict diminished survival in the very elderly[9,10]. The relative risk attached to cigarette smoking appears to diminish with advancing age in some[6,7,11], but not in all studies[8,12].

The prediction of CAD by serum cholesterol level appears to decline with advancing age[13], as indicated in Figure 1. A meta-analysis of prospective studies specifically in the elderly shows significant prediction of CAD by total cholesterol level in men, but with weaker and less consistent prediction in women[14]. This same meta-analysis has shown significant prediction of CAD by elevated low-density lipoprotein (LDL) cholesterol (men only), by

43

low levels of high-density lipoprotein (HDL) cholesterol (women only) and by elevated serum triglycerides[14].

Dubbo Study of the elderly

The Dubbo Study of the elderly is an Australian prospective study of cardiovascular disease which screened 1236 men and 1569 women in 1988–89, constituting 73% of a semirural community aged 60 years and over. This report uses data at 89-months median follow-up, by which time 350 men (28%) and 351 women (22%) had suffered a coronary outcome (ICD-9 410–414)[15–17].

The prediction of CAD by serum cholesterol level was analyzed in Dubbo in a similar way to Figure 1 and confirmed a declining ability of serum cholesterol to predict coronary disease with advancing age. The change in coronary risk per 0.6 mmol/l increase in serum cholesterol in those aged 60–64 years was 17% in men and 9% in women; in those aged

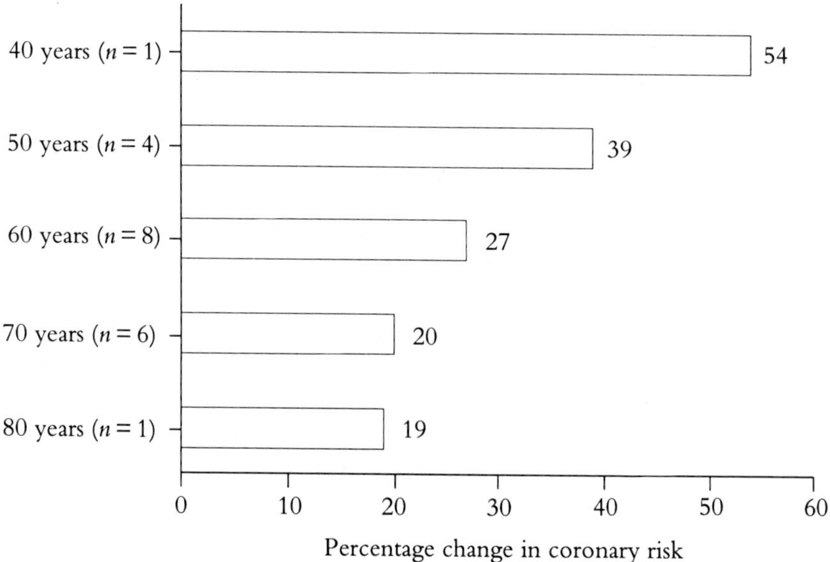

Figure 1 Percentage change in coronary risk for each 0.6 mmol/l change in serum cholesterol according to age: numbers of studies are shown in parentheses. Data modified from reference 13

65–69 years, the changes were 7% and 16% respectively. There was no significant prediction of CAD by serum cholesterol level in those of 70 years and older.

Initial versus recurrent coronary disease

Since lipid intervention studies in the elderly have largely been confined to patients with clinically manifest CAD, it would seem helpful to continue exploration of observational studies which compare initial and recurrent CAD. Lipid abnormalities remain predictive of future CAD in those who have already suffered clinical coronary disease[13]. The coronary mortality rate in the Lipid Research Clinics Prevalence Study (mean age 51 years) was much higher in those with prior cardiovascular disease (mainly coronary disease)[18]. There was an eightfold mortality gradient between total cholesterol < 5.2 mmol/l and cholesterol > 6.2 mmol/l in those with prior cardiovascular disease, compared with a fourfold gradient in mortality in those without prior cardiovascular disease[18]. Broadly similar changes were noted with respect to HDL cholesterol.

The Finnish cohort of the Seven Countries' Study included men aged 65–84 years (mean age 72 years). Each 0.6 mmol/l increase in serum cholesterol was associated with a 22% increase in risk of an initial myocardial infarction, yet only a 6% increase in risk for a recurrent myocardial infarction[19].

In the Dubbo Study, the proportion of recurrent to initial coronary events was 3:1 in men and women aged 60–69 years and 2:1 in men and women aged 70 years and older. The relationships between elevated total cholesterol (> 6.5 mmol/l), elevated LDL cholesterol (> 4.5 mmol/l) and the incidence of initial and recurrent coronary events according to age group are presented for men in Figure 2 and women in Figure 3. Hypercholesterolemia, due to excess of LDL cholesterol, was predictive of initial and recurrent CAD in men and women aged 60–69 years. The gradient of risk with LDL cholesterol was steeper for recurrent disease. Hypercholesterolemia was not consistently predictive in men and women aged 70 years and older. In a proportional hazards model in those aged 60–69 years, each 0.6 mmol/l increase in total cholesterol was associated with a 14% increase in risk of initial CAD in men and a 10% increase in women. The corresponding increases in risk for recurrent CAD were 27% and 22%

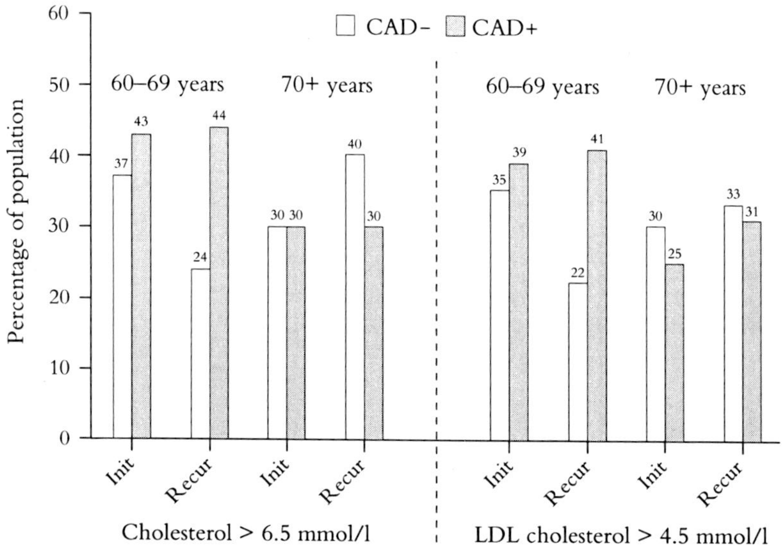

Figure 2 Relationship between elevated total or low–density lipoprotein (LDL) cholesterol and risk of coronary artery disease (CAD) in Dubbo men by age group. Those remaining free of CAD during 89-months follow-up are indicated CAD− and those developing disease are indicated CAD+. Init, initial event; Recur, recurrent event

respectively, confirming the important contribution of hypercholesterolemia to recurrent coronary disease.

In the Dubbo Study, hypertriglyceridemia (> 2.0 mmol/l) and low HDL cholesterol (< 1.0 mmol/l) were predictive of initial and recurrent CAD in men aged 60–69 years, but not older (data not presented). In women, elevated triglycerides and low HDL cholesterol were predictive in all subjects aged 60 years and older (Figure 4).

In the Dubbo Study, elevated lipoprotein(a) (> 300 mg/l) and diabetes were independently predictive of initial and recurrent CAD in men and women aged 60 years and older (data shown for women in Figure 5). The presence of antihypertensive drug therapy was predictive of CAD in both sexes at all ages (male data are shown in Figure 6). The use of any alcohol consistently predicted a reduced risk of initial and recurrent CAD in men and women aged 60–69 years, but not in older groups (Figure 6).

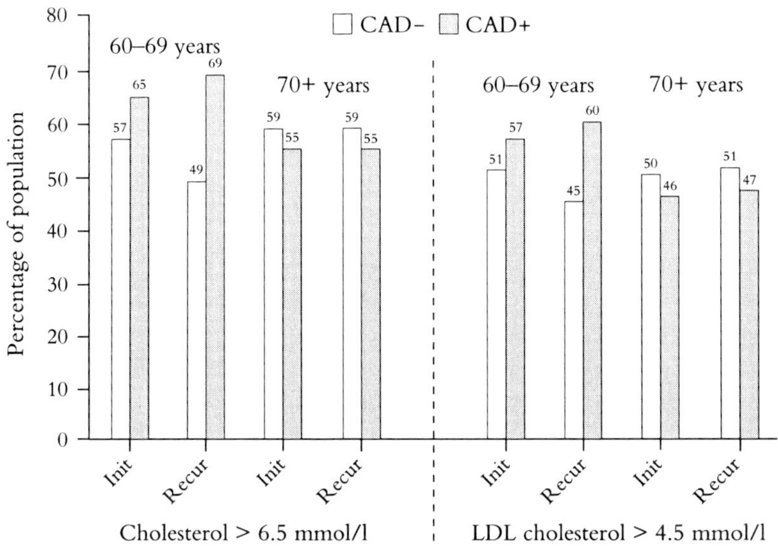

Figure 3 Relationship between elevated total or low-density lipoprotein (LDL) cholesterol and risk of coronary artery disease (CAD) in Dubbo women by age group. All symbols and abbreviations as for Figure 2

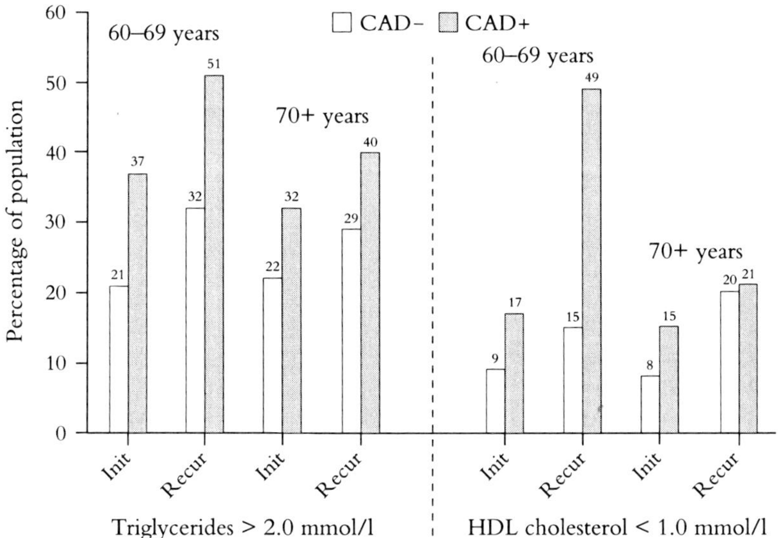

Figure 4 Relationship between elevated triglycerides or low high-density lipoprotein (HDL) cholesterol and risk of coronary artery disease (CAD) in Dubbo women by age group. All symbols and abbreviations as for Figure 2

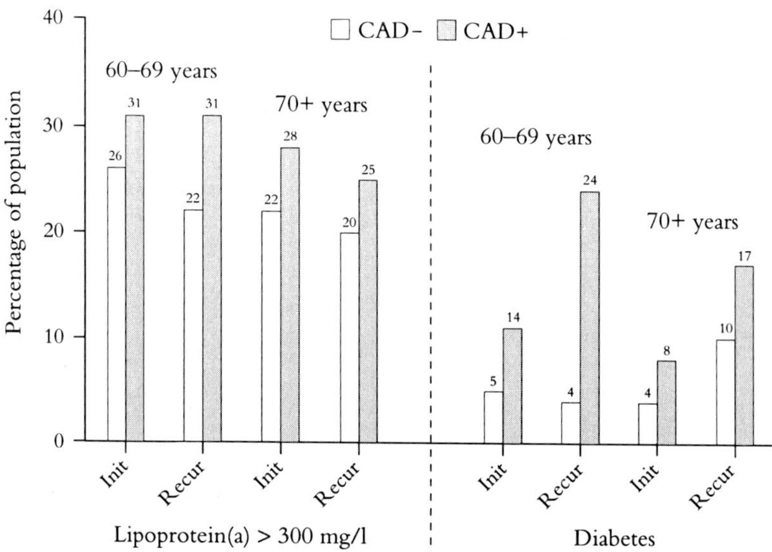

Figure 5 Relationship between elevated lipoprotein(a) or diabetes and risk of coronary artery disease (CAD) in Dubbo women by age group. All symbols and abbreviations as for Figure 2

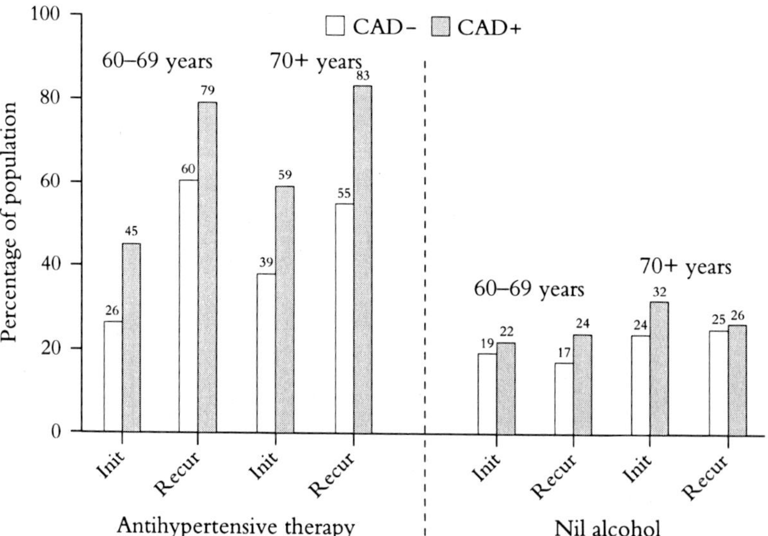

Figure 6 Relationship between use of antihypertensive drug therapy or intake of alcohol and risk of coronary artery disease (CAD) in Dubbo men by age group. All symbols and abbreviations as for Figure 2

INTERVENTIONAL STUDIES

These will be reviewed in detail by other authors and only brief comments will be made at present. Controlled trials with antihypertensive therapy clearly demonstrate coronary disease prevention in the elderly[20].

Lipid intervention trials have not been specifically conducted in elderly cohorts. A number of trials in patients with established coronary disease (or evidence of atherosclerosis) have included some subjects up to 75 years of age and certain inferences may be drawn:

(1) In the Scandinavian Simvastatin Survival Study, coronary events were reduced by 29% in men and women aged 60–69 years and by 39% in younger age groups[21].

(2) In pooled analysis of results with pravastatin, coronary events were reduced by 85% in men and women aged 65–72 years and by 55% in younger age groups[22].

(3) In the Cholesterol and Recurrent Events Trial with pravastatin in patients with 'average' cholesterol levels, coronary events were reduced by 27% in men and women aged 60–75 years and by 20% in younger age groups[23].

DISCUSSION

In the matter of lipids and CAD in the elderly, the epidemiology is conflicting and specific intervention studies notably lacking. Meta-analysis has shown that prediction of CAD by serum cholesterol level declines with advancing age[13,14]. New findings from the Dubbo Study in Australia confirm that total and LDL cholesterol levels are significant predictors of CAD in men and women aged 60–69 years, but not in still older groups. This conclusion is consistent with other studies showing no prediction in men and women aged 70 years and older[24]. The gradient of CAD risk may be steeper for recurrent disease compared with initial coronary disease in the elderly, yet even this is controversial. It has been helpful to focus on prediction of recurrent coronary disease in the elderly, since virtually all lipid intervention trials that included older subjects focused on patients with prior coronary disease.

In the Dubbo Study, low HDL cholesterol and elevated triglycerides predicted CAD in men aged 60–69 years only and in all women aged 60 years and older. This is consistent with previous meta-analysis[14] and with results from the Framingham Study, where triglycerides predicted CAD in women of 50 years and older, but not in men, and with a still higher risk in those with low HDL cholesterol[25]. Unfortunately, specific interventions targeted on elevated triglycerides or low HDL cholesterol have not been conducted in any age group.

Prospective data in the area of lipoprotein(a) and CAD remain inadequate and one cannot yet generalize in this area[17]. However, the linkage of diabetes with CAD, especially in women, has been highlighted in recent reports[26]. Excess coronary risk in the presence of antihypertensive drug therapy may appear to be a contradiction, yet this has been reported in several studies[17,27]. Earlier papers linked hypertension with CAD in the elderly[6–8], yet some studies failed to find an association[27]. This is a complex area, and it may be speculated that an increased risk of CAD in the presence of hypertension may not be fully reversible, or perhaps the treatment has been inappropriate or inadequate. Notwithstanding these comments, clinical trials in the elderly have clearly demonstrated CAD prevention by antihypertensive drug therapy[20]. A cardioprotective role for moderate alcohol intake is now generally recognized[28]. Findings in the Dubbo Study extend this observation to the elderly, where a specific survival advantage with alcohol intake was recently reported[29].

We need more basic epidemiological data in the elderly relating to risk factors for coronary disease. Similarly, lipid intervention studies in the elderly are urgently required. Meanwhile, older patients require specific management and this has to be offered on a largely inferential and empirical basis.

CONCLUSIONS RELATED TO LIPID THERAPY IN THE ELDERLY

(1) Hypercholesterolemia predicts initial and recurrent CAD in men and women aged 60–69 years, but not in older groups.

(2) Cholesterol treatment in men and women aged 60–69 years with existing CAD reduces future coronary risk.

(3) Men and women aged 60–69 years with existing CAD deserve lipid therapy. The case for lipid therapy in still older subjects with existing CAD is unresolved, but treatment may be justified on empirical grounds.

(4) The case for cholesterol therapy in subjects aged 60–69 years and free of clinical CAD remains unproven. Cholesterol therapy in those aged 70 years and older and free of CAD appears to be unjustified.

ACKNOWLEDGEMENTS

The Dubbo Study is supported by the National Health and Medical Research Council of Australia. The senior investigators are Leon Simons, John McCallum and Judith Simons in Australia and Yechiel Friedlander in Israel.

REFERENCES

1. Stokes, J., Kannel, W. B., Wolf, P. A., *et al.* (1987). The relative importance of selected risk factors for various manifestations of cardiovascular disease among men and women from 35–64 years old: 30 years of follow-up in the Framingham Study. *Circulation*, **75**, V65–V73
2. Pooling Project Research Group. (1978). Relationship of blood pressure, serum cholesterol, smoking habit, relative weight and ECG abnormalities to incidence of major coronary events: final report of the Pooling Project. *J. Chronic. Dis.*, **31**, 201–306
3. Stamler, J., Wentworth, D. and Neaton, J. D. for MRFIT Research Group. (1986). Is relationship between serum cholesterol and risk of premature death from coronary heart disease continuous and graded? Findings in 356 222 primary screenees of the Multiple Risk Factor Intervention Trial (MRFIT). *J. Am. Med. Assoc.*, **256**, 2823–8
4. Castelli, W. P., Garrison, R. J., Wilson, P. W. F., *et al.* (1986). Incidence of coronary heart disease and lipoprotein cholesterol levels: the Framingham Study. *J. Am. Med. Assoc.*, **256**, 2835–8
5. Kannel, W. B. and McGee, D. L. (1979). Diabetes and cardiovascular risk factors: the Framingham Study. *Circulation*, **59**, 8–13

6. Harris, T., Cook, E. S., Kannel, W. B., *et al.* (1988). Proportional hazards analysis of risk factors for coronary heart disease in individuals aged 65 and older: the Framingham Heart Study. *J. Am. Geriatr. Soc.*, **36**, 1023–8

7. Cullen, K., Stenhouse, N. S., Wearne, K. L., *et al.* (1983). Multiple regression analysis of risk factors for cardiovascular disease and cancer mortality in Busselton, W. A. – 13 year study. *J. Chronic. Dis.*, **36**, 371–7

8. Aronow, W. S., Herzig, A. H., Etienne, F., *et. al.* (1989). 41-months follow-up of risk factors correlated with new coronary events in 708 elderly patients. *J. Am. Geriatr. Soc.*, **37**, 501–6

9. Mattila, K., Haavisto, M., Rajala, S., *et al.* (1988). Blood pressure and survival in the very old. *Br. Med. J.*, **296**, 887–9

10. Langer, R. D., Ganiats, T. G. and Barrett-Connor, E. (1989). Paradoxical survival of elderly men with high blood pressure. *Br. Med. J.*, **298**, 1356–8

11. Benfante, R. and Reed, D. (1990). Is elevated serum cholesterol level a risk factor for coronary heart disease in the elderly? *J. Am. Med. Assoc.*, **263**, 393–6

12. Jajich, C. L., Ostfeld, A. M. and Freeman, D. H. (1984). Smoking and coronary heart disease mortality in the elderly. *J. Am. Med. Assoc.*, **252**, 2831–4

13. Law, M. R., Wald, N. J. and Thompson, G. (1994). By how much and how quickly does reduction in serum cholesterol concentration lower risk of ischaemic heart disease? *Br. Med. J.*, **308**, 367–73

14. Manolio, T. A., Pearson, T. A., Wenger, N. K., *et al.* (1992). Cholesterol and heart disease in older persons and women. Review of NHLBI Workshop. *Ann. Epidemiol.*, **2**, 161–76

15. Simons, L. A., McCallum, J., Simons, J., *et al.* (1990). The Dubbo Study: an Australian prospective community study of the health of elderly. *Aust. NZ. J. Med.*, **20**, 783–9

16. Simons, L. A., McCallum, J., Friedlander, Y., *et al.* (1991). Dubbo Study of the elderly: sociological and cardiovascular risk factors at entry. *Aust. NZ J. Med.*, **21**, 701–9

17. Simons, L. A., Friedlander, Y., McCallum, J., *et al.* (1995). Risk factors for coronary heart disease in the prospective Dubbo Study of the Australian elderly. *Atherosclerosis*, **117**, 107–18

18. Pekkanen, J., Linn, S., Heiss, G., *et al.* (1990). Ten-year mortality from cardiovascular disease in relation to cholesterol level among men with and without pre-existing cardiovascular disease. *N. Engl. J. Med.*, **322** 1700–7

19. Tervahauta, M., Pekkanen, J. and Nissinen, A. (1995). Risk factors of coronary heart disease and total mortality among elderly men with and without preexisting coronary heart disease. *J. Am. Coll. Cardiol.*, **26**, 1623–9

20. Bennet, N. E. (1994). Hypertension in the elderly. *Lancet*, **344**, 447–9
21. Scandinavian Simvastatin Survival Study Group. (1994). Randomised trial of cholesterol lowering in 4444 patients with coronary heart disease: the Scandinavian Simvastatin Survival Study (4S). *Lancet*, **344**, 1383–9
22. Byington, R. P., Jukema, J. W., Salonen, J. T., *et al.* (1995). Reduction in cardiovascular events during pravastatin therapy: pooled analysis of clinical events of the pravastatin atherosclerosis intervention program. *Circulation*, **92**, 2419–25
23. Sacks, F. M., Pfeffer, M. A., Moye, L. A., *et al.* (1996). The effect of pravastatin on coronary events after myocardial infarction in patients with average cholesterol levels. *N. Engl. J. Med.*, **335**, 1001–9
24. Krumholz, H. M., Seeman, T. E., Merrill, S. S., *et al.*, (1994). Lack of association between cholesterol and coronary heart disease mortality and morbidity and all-cause mortality in persons older than 70 years. *J. Am. Med. Assoc.*, **272**, 1335–40
25. Castelli, W. P., Wilson, P. W. F., Levy, D., *et al.* (1989). Cardiovascular risk factors in the elderly. *Am. J. Cardiol.*, **63**, 12H–19H
26. Simons, L. A., McCallum, J., Friedlander, Y., *et al.* (1996). Diabetes, mortality and coronary heart disease in the prospective Dubbo Study of Australian elderly. *Aust. NZ J. Med.*, **26**, 66–74
27. Seeman, T., Mendes de Leon, A., Berkman, L., *et al.* (1993). Risk factors for coronary heart disease among older men and women: a prospective study of community-dwelling elderly. *Am. J. Epidemiol.*, **138**, 1037–49
28. Rimm, E. B., Klatsky, A., Grobbee, D., *et al.* (1996). Review of moderate alcohol consumption and reduced risk of coronary heart disease: is the effect due to beer, wine or spirits? *Br. Med. J.*, **312**, 731–5
29. Simons, L. A., McCallum, J., Friedlander, Y., *et al.* Alcohol intake and survival in the elderly: a 77 month follow-up in the Dubbo Study. *Aust. NZ J. Med.*, **26**, 662–70

3

Cardiovascular diseases and stroke in the Asian population

Y. Goto

THE AGING PHENOMENON IN ASIA

The aging phenomenon that is affecting the world has shown the greatest impact in the Asian continent. By the year 2025, from the top ten nations worldwide with the greatest elderly (> 60 years old) population, six will be Asian countries: the People's Republic of China (1st), India (2nd), Japan (5th), Indonesia (7th), Pakistan (8th) and Bangladesh (10th) (Table 1).

The aging process accentuates the increase in the incidence of chronic, degenerative diseases such as cardiovascular diseases, stroke and cancer, and, as will be discussed in this chapter, the process is particularly noticeable in the Asian countries.

Table 1   Countries with more than 16 million elderly by the year 2025

Country	*People above 60 years of age* ($\times$ *1 million*)			
	1975	*2000*	*2025*	*Position*
China	73	134	284	1st
India	29	65	146	2nd
EC	34	54	71	3rd
USA	31	40	67	4th
Japan	13	26	33	5th
Brazil	6	14	32	6th
Indonesia	7	15	31	7th
Pakistan	3	7	18	8th
Mexico	3	6	17	9th
Bangladesh	3	6	17	10th

CAUSES OF DEATH IN ASIAN COUNTRIES[1]

Information with regard to the mortality rate due to cardiovascular diseases and stroke in various Asian countries is well documented. However, there is a relative lack of information when it is those rates specifically among the elderly which are required. This is due in part to the fact that, although the incidence of cardiovascular diseases, mainly ischemic heart disease, is increasing in Asia, since the incidence was low until some years ago, there were few epidemiologic studies considering cardiovascular and cerebro-vascular diseases as the main end-points for the studies in many Asian countries.

Heart diseases and cerebrovascular diseases are among the three leading causes of death in: Brunei, Hong Kong, Indonesia, Israel, Japan, Korea, Kuwait, Malaysia, the People's Republic of China, the Philippines, Singapore, Sri Lanka, Taiwan and Thailand (Table 2). Heart diseases are the main cause of death in: Brunei, Indonesia, Israel, Malaysia, the Philippines and Thailand. As 'heart diseases' include different cardiovascular diseases, it is believed that, in many of those countries, rheumatic heart diseases are more prevalent than ischemic heart diseases as the cause of death.

The second cause of death in Singapore is heart disease, and in Taiwan and Japan it is cerebrovascular disease. The main cause of death in both countries is cancer. Other second causes of death are: malignant neoplasms in Israel, accidents, poisoning and other violence in Brunei and Thailand, tuberculosis in Indonesia, pneumonia in the Philippines and perinatal diseases in Malaysia.

Table 2 Leading causes of death in some Asian countries

Country	1st	2nd	3rd	4th
Brunei	Heart	Accidents	Cancer	Stroke
Indonesia	Heart	Tuberculosis	Pneumonia	Diarrhea
Israel	Heart	Cancer	Stroke	Pneumonia
Japan	Cancer	Stroke	Heart	Pneumonia
Malaysia	Heart	Perinatal	Stroke	Stroke
Philippines	Heart	Pneumonia	Stroke	Cancer
Singapore	Cancer	Heart	Stroke	Pneumonia
Taiwan	Cancer	Stroke	Accidents	Heart
Thailand	Heart	Accidents	Cancer	Stroke

Heart diseases are the third cause of death in Japan, cerebrovascular diseases are the third cause of death in Israel, Malaysia, Singapore and the Philippines. The third cause of death in other countries includes: malignant neoplasms in Brunei and Thailand, accidents in Taiwan and respiratory infection in Indonesia.

Cerebrovascular diseases are the fourth cause of death in Brunei, Thailand and Sarawak in Malaysia. In other countries, as the fourth cause of death, we have: cancer in the Philippines, heart diseases in Taiwan, pneumonia in Israel, Japan and Singapore, and diarrhea in Indonesia.

What is worth noting is that the infectious diseases are giving place to the degenerative disorders as the main causes of death in almost all Asian countries.

Japan

In Japan, from the 1960s until the late 1970s, cerebrovascular diseases were the leading cause of death. During the 1980s, malignant neoplasms became the first cause of death among the Japanese people, and from the mid 1980s, heart diseases became the second and cerebrovascular diseases the third cause of death. Eleven years later, in 1995, cerebrovascular diseases again became the second cause of death with heart diseases the third (Figure 1).

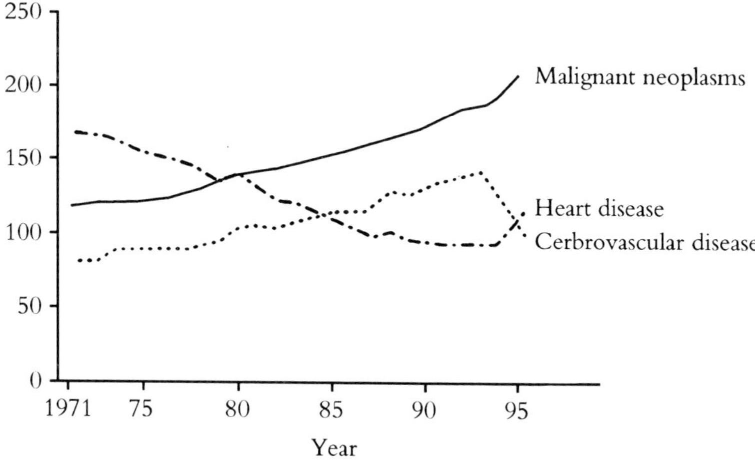

Figure 1   Trends in the three leading causes of death in Japan

The Philippines

For many years, pneumonia was the main cause of death in the Philippines. However, since 1990, heart diseases became the leading cause of death followed by pneumonia, vascular diseases and cancer (Figure 2).

Malaysia

The peninsular of Malaysia has had heart diseases and diseases of the pulmonary circulation as the main causes of death for many years. Perinatal diseases are now the second cause of death and cerebrovascular diseases, the third (Figure 3).

Thailand

In Thailand, from the 1930s to the 1950s, the leading cause of death was malaria. Between 1970 and 1980 it was accidents and during the 1980s, heart diseases and diseases of pulmonary circulation were the main causes of death. From 1992, diseases of the heart are the first cause of death followed by: accidents and poisoning, malignant neoplasms, hypertension and cerebrovascular diseases (Figure 4).

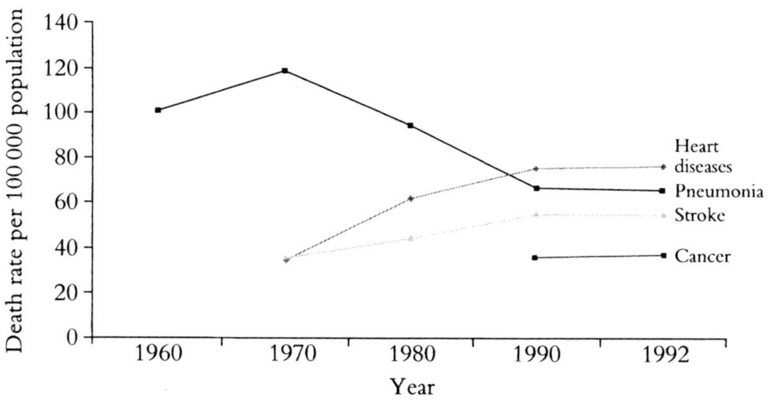

Figure 2   Trends in the leading causes of death in the Philippines

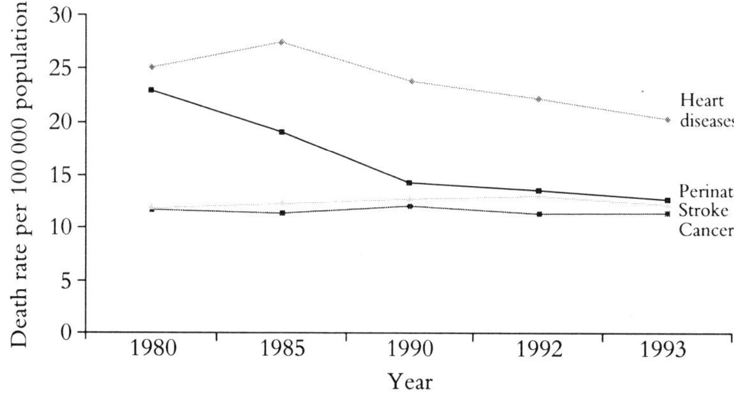

Figure 3   Trends in the leading causes of death in Malaysia

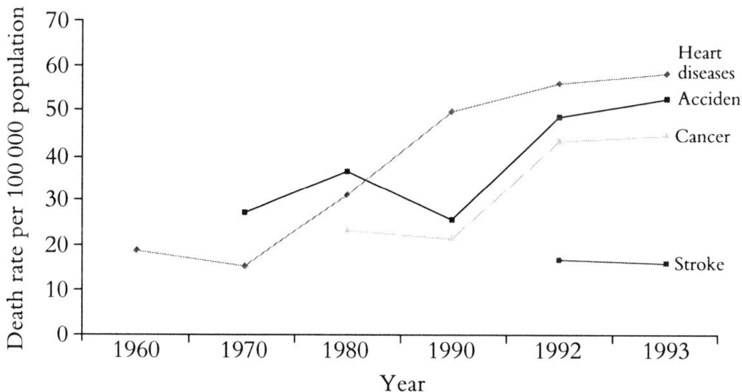

Figure 4   Trends in the leading causes of death in Thailand

Singapore[2]

Until the 1950s, the major causes of death in Singapore were tuberculosis, gastroenteritis, pneumonia and various childhood infections. During the 1960s and 1970s, cancer became the main cause of death in Singapore. During the 1980s, heart diseases became the first cause of death and, in the 1990s, cancer reassumed the first position as cause of death, followed by heart diseases and cerebrovascular diseases (Figure 5).

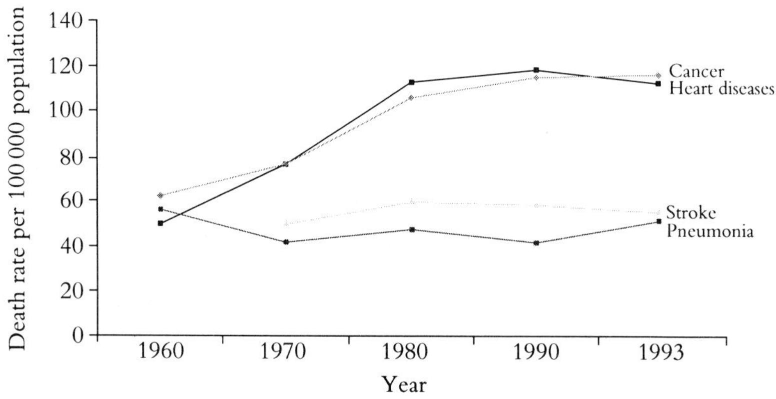

Figure 5   Trends in the leading causes of death in Singapore

Heart diseases and cancer, the two major killers of Singaporeans, each account for approximately 25 per cent of deaths. Among the heart diseases, ischemic heart diseases are the more prevalent. The mortality rate from ischemic heart disease is greatest among the Indian population, their rate being about twice that of the Malays and Chinese in Singapore. The heart disease rate is now 120 per 100 000 Singaporeans. Singapore has overtaken Australia in having the highest mortality rate from ischemic heart disease in the eastern Pacific.

Aging of the population

Singapore has the second fastest-growing, aging society in the world and this fact aggravates the heart disease problem. It is already known that aging is one of the most powerful risk factors for heart diseases. The average life-span of Singaporean women is 77 years, and Singaporean men, 73 years.

Change in the dietary habits

From 1960 until 1985, the percentage of calories from fat in the diet of the Singaporeans increased enormously, consumption of meat and offal increased 135 per cent and egg consumption increased 80 per cent.

Sedentarism, obesity and smoking

Physical activity from 1960 to 1985 decreased in women while the incidence of obesity increased, and smoking increased from 1960 to 1977.

The average serum cholesterol level in adult Singaporeans without clinical evidence of myocardial ischemia is now 228 mg/dl (5.9 mmol/l) and among those with clinical evidence of myocardial ischemia, 239 mg/dl (6.2 mmol/l). These levels rank Singaporeans fifth highest in the world: only Finland, Norway, the United Kingdom and Germany have higher levels. Among Singaporean adults, 55 per cent have serum total cholesterol levels above 200 mg/dl (5.2 mmol/l) and 27 per cent of Singaporeans have levels above 250 mg/dl (6.5 mmol/l).

In adult Singaporeans, with and without clinical evidence of myocardial ischemia, low-density lipoprotein (LDL) cholesterol averages 163 mg/dl, high-density lipoprotein (HDL) cholesterol, 39 mg/dl, and the total cholesterol to HDL-cholesterol ratio, 6.3. The serum triglyceride levels are usually below 160 mg/dl (2.1 mmol/l).

From the data presented on the trend of the leading causes of death and of the cardiovascular risk factors in Singapore, we can clearly note that there is an unequivocal increase in the prevalence of heart diseases with the worsening of the risk factors profile of the population.

India[3]

As in all developing countries, rheumatic fever and rheumatic heart disease are common in India. Systemic hypertension however is not as common as it is in the western world. It is estimated that about 5 per cent of its population above 20 years of age have systemic arterial blood pressure above 140/90 mmHg. Five per cent of 400 million still amounts to 20 million people.

It is a little surprising that ischemic heart disease is as common as it is in India. The reason seems to be the abundance of very saturated fat in the diet. Although the meat of the cow is rarely eaten in India, milk and butter, rich in saturated fat, are consumed freely, and in spite of the fact that many Hindus are vegetarians, coconut oil, which is 92 per cent saturated fat, is the most common fatty acid consumed in India, presumably because it is relatively cheap. Chicken meat is by far the most common meat consumed in India, but the chicken fat is also eaten, not discarded. This intake of saturated fatty acids is probably one of the reasons for the incidence of ischemic heart diseases in India.

China[4,5]

Stroke is the second most common cause of death among urban residents and the third most common cause of death in rural residents of the People's Republic of China (China). Each year, stroke accounts for over 1 million deaths in China, more than three times the number of deaths from ischemic heart disease.

In the World Health Organization Multi-international Monitoring of Trends and Determinants in Cardiovascular Disease (MONICA) project, the incidence of ischemic heart diseases in China was the lowest among the 42 populations studied, but the incidence of stroke was higher in China than in most of the other populations.

There are two interesting characteristics regarding stroke in China: first is the type of stroke and second is the geographical distribution. First, regarding the type of stroke, it is known that the pathological patterns of stroke in China are different from those noted in most western populations. Hemorrhagic stroke is as common as ischemic stroke in China, whereas cerebral infarction is the predominant cause of stroke in most western populations. Second, regarding the geographical distribution of stroke, it is known that there is a north to south gradient, with a significantly higher incidence and mortality of stroke in the north compared with the south.

The analysis of Chinese Stroke and Hypertension Surveys shows that, among the known risk factors for stroke:

- hypertension may account for about half of all deaths from stroke in China. A 10 per cent increase in the prevalence of hypertension was associated with a 2.8-fold higher incidence and 2.68-fold higher mortality from stroke.

- a 10 per cent increase in the prevalence of alcohol consumption was associated with a 29 per cent higher incidence and a 16 per cent higher mortality from stroke.

- a 10 per cent in the prevalence of cigarette smoking was associated with a 19 per cent higher mortality from stroke.

With regard to this excess risk of stroke associated with hypertension in China, some investigators have suggested that blood pressure is more strongly related to stroke in populations with a lower level of serum cholesterol. On average, the serum cholesterol levels of the Chinese population are much lower than those in most western populations. The lower serum cholesterol levels may also partially explain why the proportion of hemorrhagic stroke is much higher in China than in western populations. It is known that higher levels of serum cholesterol may be protective against hemorrhagic stroke. In addition, mean body mass is much lower in China than in western populations. There are data showing that the risk of hemorrhagic stroke associated with hypertension is greater in people of low body weight. Moreover, dietary differences, such as lower dietary protein and higher salt intake in China compared with western countries, may also contribute to the higher risk of stroke related to hypertension. Lower dietary protein and higher salt intake have been associated with an increased risk of hypertension and stroke.

Dr Cheng and colleagues' data[4] show that there has been an apparent decline in stroke incidence in recent years. Marked differences in rates were found between males and females with a decline in incidence occurring almost exclusively in males. These differences may result in part from differences in diet, alcohol and cigarette consumption, or prevalence of hypertension and its treatment in the cities studied (Figure 6).

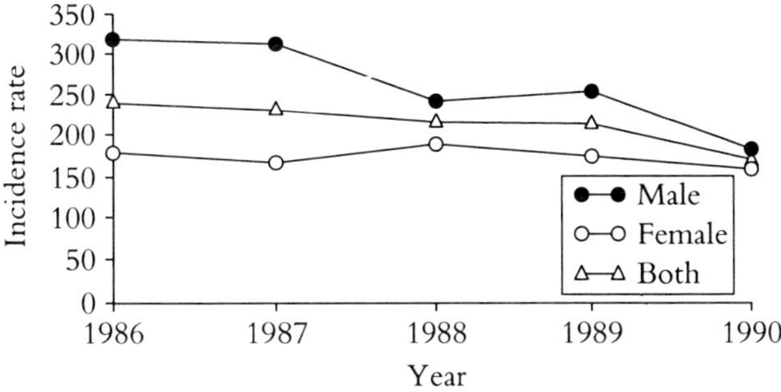

Figure 6   Stroke in China – effects of intervention

CARDIOVASCULAR DISEASES AND STROKE IN ASIAN COUNTRIES

MONICA Project[6]

During the 1980s, the World Health Organization developed the MONICA project surveying the incidence of stroke and myocardial infarction around the world. As there were no Japanese data in the MONICA study, Professor Fukiyama, from Ryukyu University, calculated the matched incidence rates for stroke and myocardial infarction for the same age–range population (35 to 64 years of age) from Okinawa, adjusting for the normalized world population. The age-adjusted incidence rate of stroke in Okinawa is:

- comparable to the incidence in Warsaw (Poland);

- lower than that in northern Sweden, Glostrup (Denmark), Novi Sad (Yugoslavia), three different regions of Finland, Kaunas (Lithuania), Moscow (Russia), and Beijing (China); and

- a little higher than in Goteborg (Sweden), Rhein-Necker (Germany), and Friuli (Italy).

With regard to myocardial infarction, the age-adjusted incidence rate of myocardial infarction in Okinawa is considerably lower than in American, European or Oceanian countries and slightly lower than the incidence in Beijing, China.

As there are no large differences in the incidence rates of stroke and myocardial infarction from Okinawa and from other regions of Japan, regarding the incidence of circulatory diseases we can say that, in Japan:

- contrary to western countries, the incidence of stroke is higher than that of myocardial infarction;

- the incidence of stroke is high, however not astronomically high compared to other nations, as was once believed;

- the incidence of myocardial infarction is much lower than in western countries.

CARDIOVASCULAR DISEASES AND STROKE IN JAPAN[8,9]

The great majority of countries have shown a decrease in the death rate from stroke in the period from 1970 to 1992 and it is worth noting that Japan, which had the highest death rate in the world from stroke in the early 1970s, presented a dramatic decrease compared to the rate among the developed countries, which is still high.

When considering the trends in the death rates from ischmeic heart diseases, it is clear that Japan, together with China, always presented the lowest rates of deaths.

With regard to women's data for both cerebrovascular and ischemic heart diseases, although the rates are lower than those for men, the trends from 1970 to 1992 are similar.

Regarding the incidence of stroke and myocardial infarction in the elderly (above 65 years of age) in Japan[10,11], for both men and women, the incidence rate of stroke increases with age, with highest rates above 85 years. It is notable that while the incidence rate for stroke increases with age, that of myocardial infarction does not change significantly with age, and continues at very low rates as for the younger age ranges.

Data from a comparison study of incidence rates of stroke and myocardial infarction between Japan (Okinawa) and the USA (Rochester) give us interesting information[10,11]. While in Rochester the incidence of myocardial infarction is higher than that of stroke, in Okinawa, the incidence rate of stroke is much higher than that of myocardial infarction. It is worth noting the very low incidence of myocardial infarction in Okinawa compared to that of Rochester.

The incidence rates of stroke do not show significant differences between the two regions and, in both regions, there is a common tendency for an increase in incidence after 70 years of age.

While the incidence rate of myocardial infarction shows a clear increase with age in Rochester, in Okinawa, this age-dependency is not so clear, showing a kind of 'plateau' after 70 years of age.

RISK FACTORS FOR ASYMPTOMATIC LACUNAR INFARCTION[12]

Dr Takagi from the Department of Neurology of Tokai University, Japan, conducted a study searching for asymptomatic lacunar infarction in subjects without clinical manifestations of cerebrovascular diseases.

For this purpose, the team performed brain magnetic resonance imaging (MRI), looking for lacunar infarction, in 882 men with a mean age of 51 ± 10 years and 376 women with a mean age of 53 ± 10 years, with no manifestation of cerebrovascular diseases.

From 882 male participants, 87 showed asymptomatic cerebral infarction, 84 (9.5 per cent) presenting with lacunar infarction. Fifteen cases presented with suspicion for lacunar infarction and there was 1 case of asymptomatic cerebral bleeding (Table 3). Of the 376 female participants, 22 (5.6 per cent) presented with lacunar infarction and there were 6 cases with suspicion for lacunar infarction.

The mean age of the 84 male participants with asymptomatic lacunar infarction was 59 ± 9 years, significantly higher ($p < 0.0001$) than the mean age of the 779 male controls, with a mean age of 50 ± 10 years. In the same way, the mean age of the 22 female participants with asymptomatic lacunar infarction was 58 ± 11 years, significantly higher ($p < 0.05$) than the mean age of the 348 female controls with a mean age of 52 ± 10 years.

There was a clear correlation between the frequency of the asymptomatic lacunar infarction and the age. In men, there were 1/113 cases (0.9 per cent) of lacunar infarction below 39 years, 11/283 (3.9 per cent) in the 40s, 28/309 (9.1 per cent) in the 50s, 36/155 (23.2 per cent) in the 60s and 8/22 (36.4 per cent) above 70 years of age, showing a clear increase in the rate of lacunar

Table 3 Factors for asymptomatic lacunar infarction

	Male		*Female*	
	Lacunar	*Control*	*Lacunar*	*Control*
N	84	779	22	348
Age	59 ± 9**	59 ± 10	58 ± 11*	52 ± 10
Systolic BP	138 ± 17**	130 ± 17	132 ± 17*	125 ± 20
Diastolic BP	84 ± 12*	80 ± 11	79 ± 13	76 ± 12
Mean BP	102 ± 13**	97 ± 13	97 ± 14	92 ± 15

*$p < 0.05$ vs. control; **$p < 0.0001$ vs. control

infarction with age. In the same way, in women, there were 1/30 cases (3.3 per cent) of lacunar infarction below 39 years, 4/113 (3.5 per cent) in the 40s, 8/143 (5.6 per cent) in the 50s, 6/75 (8.0 per cent) in the 60s and 3/15 (20.0 per cent) above 70 years of age, showing a clear increase in the rate of lacunar infarction with age.

It is interesting to note the impact of blood pressure on this increase in the rate of lacunar infarction with age. In the group with normal blood pressure, the incidence of lacunar infarction was 6 per cent or less in the 50s and a little above 20 per cent in the 60s. However, in the group with systolic blood pressure above 140 mmHg or diastolic blood pressure above 90 mmHg or mean blood pressure above 107 mmHg, the incidence of lacunar infarction was around 20 per cent already in the 50s, showing that in the hypertensive subjects lacunar infarction would start 10 years earlier when compared to normotensive controls.

SERUM CHOLESTEROL LEVEL IN THE JAPANESE POPULATION[13–15]

In 1980 and 1990, the national survey on circulatory disorder was conducted in Japan, as the annual Japanese Nutrition Survey, to determine the prevalence of risk factors for cardiovascular diseases. Between 1980 and 1990, age-adjusted serum cholesterol levels increased from 186 to 201 mg/dl for men and from 189 to 202 mg/dl for women. Energy supply from dietary fat increased from 23.4 to 25.1 per cent.

The comparison of average adult cholesterol levels between Japan and the USA in 1990 shows them to be extremely close.

CHANGES IN STROKE INCIDENCE, MORTALITY AND RISK FACTORS IN THE ELDERLY JAPANESE POPULATION (HISAYAMA TOWN STUDY)[16]

For several decades, Japan has experienced a great change in dietary and living patterns[17,18], which may have an effect on stroke morbidity and mortality, and their risk factors. Thus, to determine the basis of the change in stroke death, changes in incidence and risk factors for stroke were examined in the general population of Hisayama Town, where a prospective population survey of cerebrovascular disease was initiated in 1961[19].

Hisayama Town is located in the neighborhood of Fukuoka City, a metropolitan area on Kyushu Island in Japan. The population of the town is about 7000, and its age and occupational composition have been typical of those of the general population of Japan during the past 30 years[19, 20].

Dr Fujishima established three cohort studies of Hisayama residents free from stroke and myocardial infarction aged 40 years or over in 1961 (1618 men and women, early or first cohort), in 1974 (2047 subjects, mid or second cohort) and in 1983 (2460 subjects, recent cohort). All cohort studies included more than 80 per cent of residents of the same age range.

When considering the age-adjusted mortality from major causes of death during each 13-year follow-up period for the early and mid cohort, autopsy rates were similar in both cohorts (82.0 and 86.1 per cent, respectively). In the early cohort from 1961 to 1974, the leading cause of death was stroke, and the mortality rate was 5.6 per 1000 person-years, which was followed by death from malignancy (5.5) and heart disease (3.0). In the mid cohort from 1974 to 1987, stroke mortality rate was markedly decreased to 2.5 per 1000 person-years, or less than 50 per cent of the early cohort. In contrast, the number of deaths from malignancy increased but its age-adjusted mortality rate remained unchanged. Death rate from heart disease was slightly but significantly decreased from 3.0 per 1000 person-years in the early cohort to 2.3 in the mid cohort. Among heart diseases, however, mortality rate from myocardial infarction was very low (0.8% and 0.9%) and did not change between the two cohorts. It was recognized that the mortality rate for stroke was much higher than that for heart disease in the early cohort and also slightly higher in the mid cohort in Hisayama.

The all-cause mortality rates between the early and mid cohorts were compared by age. Mortality decreased significantly in the mid cohort compared with the early cohort both in subjects aged $\geq$ 60 years ($p < 0.001$) and in those aged < 60 years ($p < 0.01$). The difference was larger in the elderly subjects, suggesting that stroke mortality has decreased in recent years, especially in the elderly.

SILENT MYOCARDIAL ISCHEMIA IN THE ELDERLY[21]

To elucidate the clinical features of acute myocardial infarction (AMI) and silent myocardial ischemia (SMI) in the elderly, and the efficacy of therapy in an era of coronary intervention, a total of 10 607 patients with AMI who were enrolled in a multicenter survey between 1982 and 1992 were examined.

The elderly had a higher ratio of females, non-cardiac illness, atypical symptoms at the onset of AMI, severe pump failure at admission, cardiac rupture and multivessel disease. Hospital mortality was markedly higher in patients $\geq$ 75 years, and it was 4-fold compared with patients < 65 years. In the last 5 years, the rate of application of coronary angiography and primary percutaneous transluminal coronary angioplasty (PTCA) significantly increased even in the very old. In contrast, use of thrombolysis greatly diminished.

Dr Nakahara[22], Tokyo Metropolitan Geriatric Hospital, reported that, among 770 consecutive autopsies, death due to myocardial infarction was more frequent in asymptomatic cardiac patients than in those with angina or cerebrovascular disease; problems doing activities of daily living, and communication disturbance were also more common in asymptomatic patients than in those with angina.

IMPACT OF CHANGES IN LIFESTYLE ON THE INCIDENCE OF CARDIOVASCULAR DISEASES AND STROKE IN ASIAN COUNTRIES

In conclusion, on the subject of cardiovascular diseases and stroke in Asian populations, some considerations should be made of the impact of the changes in lifestyle of the Asian countries on the incidence of heart diseases and stroke.

It is interesting to note that the proportion of heart diseases to stroke in Asian countries is different from that of western countries. While in the western countries the incidence of heart diseases is typically higher than that of stroke, in many of the Asian countries, this ratio tends to favor a higher incidence of stroke. Even inside Asia, this heart disease to stroke ratio presents a kind of gradient from the eastern side (China, Taiwan, Korea and Japan) where the stroke incidence is higher, to the western side (Israel, Kuwait) where the incidence of heart diseases is higher than that of stroke.

This phenomenon seems to reflect the impact of lifestyle, mainly diet, on the incidence of diseases. The case of Hong Kong which, although in

China, presents a higher incidence of heart diseases than stroke, may be an example of how lifestyle can influence the incidence of diseases.

There is no doubt that the incidence of heart diseases and stroke increases exponentially with aging. The morbidity and mortality related to heart diseases and stroke in the elderly have a great impact on the costs of the healthcare system and on the quality of life of the entire society.

Differences in the prevalence and treatment of risk factors for heart diseases and stroke, such as hypertension, hypercholesterolemia, cigarette smoking and alcohol consumption, as well as differences in mean dietary protein and lipid intake, may all play a role in the incidence of cardiovascular diseases and stroke. The management of those risk factors and lifestyles may be vital for the future, not only of Asian society, but also of the world.

REFERENCES

1. SEAMIC Health Statistics 1994
2. Roberts, W. C. (1991). From the Editor: Singapore and Singaporean cardiology. *Am. J. Cardiol.*, **67**, 298–1302
3. Roberts, W. C. (1988). From the Editor: India and Indian cardiology. *Am. J. Cardiol.*, **62**, 1326–9
4. Cheng, S. M., Ziegler, D. K., Lai, Y. H., *et al.* (1995). Stroke incidence in China, 1986 through 1990. *Stroke*, **26**, 1990–4
5. He, J., Klag, M. J., Wu, Z. *et al.* (1995). Stroke in people's republic of China: I. Geographic variations in incidence and risk factors. *Stroke*, **26**, 2222–7
6. Asplund, K., Bonita, R., Kuulasmaa, K. *et al.* (1995). Multinational comparisons of stroke epidemiology: evaluation of case ascertainment in the WHO stroke MONICA Study. *Stroke*, **26**, 355–60
7. Tunstal, P. H., Kuulasmaa, K., Amouyel, P. *et al.* (1994). Myocardial infarction and coronary deaths in the World Health Organization MONICA project: registration procedures, event rates, and case fatality rates in 38 populations from 21 countries in four continents. *Circulation*, **90**, 583–612
8. National Heart, Lung and Blood Institute: Annual Report Fiscal Year 1995, Report on International Activities, October 1, 1994–Septmeber 30, 1995
9. Lee, T. K., Huang, Z. S., Ng, S. K., *et al.* (1995). Impact of alcohol consumption and cigarette smoking on stroke among the elderly in Taiwan. *Stroke*, **26**, 790–4

10. Fukiyama, K. (1996). Hypertension and cardiovascular diseases in Japanese elderly. *Jpn. J. Geriat*, **33**, 335–9 (in Japanese)

11. Fukiyama, K. (1996). Trend in variation of incidence of cardiovascular disease. *Rinsho Seijin-byo*, **26**, 1056–61 (in Japanese)

12. Takagi, S., Ide, M., Yasuda, S., *et al.* (1996). Risk factors for asymptomatic lacunar infarction in subjects without symptomatic cerebrovascular disease. *Jpn. J. Stroke*, **18**, 85–92 (in Japanese)

13. Research committee on atherosclerosis in Japan. (1965). Total serum cholesterol levels in normal subjects in Japan. *Jpn. Circul. J.*, **29**, 505–10 (in Japanese)

14. Research committee on atherosclerosis in Japan. (1973). Total serum cholesterol and triglyceride levels in normal subjects in Japan. *Jpn. J. Atherosclerosis*, **1**, 101–8 (in Japanese)

15. Research Committee on Serum Lipid Level Survey. (1996). Current state of and recent trends in serum lipid levels in the general Japanese population. *J. Atheroscl. Thromb.*, **2**, 122–32

16. Fujishima, M. (1996). Changes in stroke incidence, mortality and risk factors in elderly Japanese. In Kawashima, Y., Omae, T., Lakatta, E. G. eds. (1996). *Stroke mortality and risk factors*. New York: Churchill Livingstone, 205–15

17. Fujishima, M., *et al.* (1992). Smoking as cardiovascular risk factor in low cholestrol population: the Hisayama study. *Clin. Exp. Hypertens.*, **14**, 99–108

18. Kato, I., *et al.* (1993). Serum lipids and nutritional intake in a Japanese general population: the Hisayama study. *Ann. NY Acad. Sci.*, **676**, 331–3

19. Katsuki, S. (1996). Epidemiological and clinicopathological study on cerebrovascular disease in Japan. *Prog. Brain Res.*, **21B**, 64–89

20. Ohmura, T., *et al.* (1993). Prevalence of type 2 (non-insulin-dependent) diabetes mellitus and impaired glucose tolerance in the Japanese general population: the Hisayama study. *Diabetologia*, **36**, 1198–203

21. Haze, K., Oka, T., Sumiyoshi, T., *et al.* (1996). Acute myocardial infarction and silent myocardial ischemia in the elderly – clinical features and effectiveness of therapy in an era of coronary intervention. *Jpn. J. Geriat*, **33**, 346–52 (in Japanese)

22. Nakahara, K., Matsushita, S., Yamanouchi, H., *et al.* (1997). Relation of asymptomatic myocardial ischemia to impaired communication, cerebrovascular disease, and lack of ability to perform activities of daily living in elderly patients. *Jpn. J. Geriat*, **34**, 285–91 (in Japanese)

4

Women, menopause and the primary prevention of cardiovascular disease

R. Bonita

INTRODUCTION

Cardiovascular disease (CVD) is the leading cause of death and disability in postmenopausal women in both developing and developed countries. In most industrialized countries, CVD mortality rates have been declining for several decades in women, as in men, and in all age groups; for stroke there has been an acceleration of this trend since the early 1970s. Most of the postponed deaths have occurred in older people (75 years and over). Women have benefited more than men in these favorable trends and this is reflected in the continuing gap in life expectancy between men and women.

The benefits of antihypertensive treatment have been established in randomized controlled trials for the general hypertensive population, but the magnitude of the benefit is less for preventing coronary events than stroke. This is particularly true for women, in whom most reported studies have shown no decrease in the incidence of CVD with antihypertensive treatment. It appears that much of the decline is due to factors other than antihypertensive treatment including favorable trends in smoking, cholesterol levels, exercise, and dietary changes. Conversely, where the trends in major risk factors for CVD are in a negative direction, as in many countries in central and eastern Europe, increases in CVD mortality have been noted.

While heart disease is increasingly depicted as linked to the menopause, there is no immediate increase in incidence at menopause. In the third and fourth decades after menopause, however, as with men, there is a rapid increase in CVD risk. Hormone use for menopausal women has become a widespread form of treatment for the prevention of heart disease on the basis of observational studies that may be subject to bias; its effectiveness in

73

preventing vascular disease is yet to be established in large randomized controlled trials.

A rational prevention and control policy for CVD includes the primary prevention of hypertension and smoking control directed towards the whole population. Strategies directed at individual women require treatment decisions based on absolute risk of a CVD event. It is clear that CVD can be prevented or postponed to a marked degree. Research on specific preventive strategies for older women have lagged behind the focus on menopausal women despite the fact that older women are at a greater absolute risk of CVD than pre- or perimenopausal women.

The global cardiovascular burden in women

The common view is that cardiovascular disease (CVD) is a men's health problem. This has overshadowed the recognition of the significance of CVD for women's health. Coronary heart disease (CHD) and stroke are two leading causes of death in women globally. Each year, of the 24 million deaths in women, 7.4 million are attributed to CVD, with almost two-thirds occurring in developing countries. In absolute numbers, there are more deaths in women attributed to CVD than in men. As death from cardiovascular diseases is frequently preceded by a period of morbidity and disability, heart disease and stroke also account for a high proportion of disability. It is projected that the current ranking of Disability Adjusted Life Years (DALYS) for CHD and stroke, now 4th and 6th in women, will shift to 2nd and 3rd place respectively by 2020[1].

Worldwide, 83% of all CVD deaths in women occur at older ages, 60 years and above. Already more than half the world's women aged 60 years and over live in developing regions: 149 million compared to 121 million in developed regions. The future growth in the numbers and proportion of aging women in developing countries is foreshadowed in the distribution of those now aged 45–59 years. Two-thirds of the women in this age group, 213 million, live in developing countries and only one-third, 98 million, live in developed countries.

Life expectancy at birth for women is projected to increase in all regions of the world such that by the year 2020 the life expectancy in women will reach 87–90 years in wealthy countries and 67 years even in the poorest countries[1]. The diseases of early childhood will be traded for chronic diseases, particularly CVD, in old age[2]. Increasing longevity will result in a corresponding increase in the incidence, prevalence and disability due to cardiovascular diseases in older women – and men – in the coming years unless preventive measures compensate for demographic trends. However, even small reductions in the incidence of CHD and stroke will result in fewer new cardiovascular events in the future despite the increase in the older population.

International differences and trends in CVD mortality

Unfortunately, information on mortality is limited to about one-third of the world's population. Data provided to the World Health Organization (WHO) by member nations indicate that there is a wide variation in both CHD and stroke mortality rates between countries. Age standardized CHD mortality rates vary widely, with a 12-fold difference between the country with the highest rate, Scotland (166.7 per 100 000), and the country with the lowest rate, Japan (13.1 per 100 000). In all countries, CHD rates are 2- to 5-fold higher in men than in women (Table 1). The pattern is similar for stroke mortality, and the difference in the country with the highest rate, Bulgaria (154 per 100 000), and the country with the lowest rate, Switzerland (16 per 100 000) is > 9-fold. The stroke mortality ratio between men and women is less than 2 to 1.

Table 1 Age-standardized coronary heart disease (CHD) mortality rates (per 100 000 population) in 1993, percentage change per annum 1970–1993 in women aged 40–69 years in 10 selected countries, and ratio of men to women

Country	Rate, 1993	% change 1970–1993	Ratio men/women
UK: Scotland	166.7	−1.7	2.6
Hungary	141.8	+0.6	3.1
Singapore	117.8	+2.0	2.3
Romania	114.1	+3.5	2.5
UK: England/Wales	106.4	−1.2	3.1
USA	87.2	−4.4	2.8
Finland	81.0	−3.3	4.7
Australia	70.6	−5.3	3.2
Canada	66.5	−4.2	3.3
Japan	13.1	−5.1	3.1

Substantial declines in CVD mortality rates in some, but not all, countries during the past few decades have occurred in both men and women, indicating the extent of improvement that can be achieved. The decline has been as much as 5% per annum in Australia and Japan. Not all countries have benefited from these favorable trends; the notable exceptions are central and eastern European countries and Singapore (Table 1). The reduction in stroke mortality has been even steeper; for example, the decline in stroke in Japan has been 7% per annum for the period 1970–1993. In the majority of developed countries for which trend data are available, women have benefited more than men in these favorable trends and this is reflected in the continuing gap in life expectancy at older ages between men and women.

Explanations for these trends are currently under investigation, in particular, the multinational collaborative study co-ordinated by WHO which is monitoring the trends and determinants of cardiovascular disease (the MONICA Project) in 32 countries using standard methodology[3]. Declines in mortality could be related to a decline in incidence, suggesting successful primary prevention, a decline in case fatality, suggesting improved management and treatment after the event, or a combination of both[4]. Much of the improvement in mortality has been attributed to substantial changes in population levels of risk factors.

CVD risk factors

There is abundant evidence that the standard modifiable risk factors for CVD – a diet in saturated fat which leads to above optimal levels of blood cholesterol, cigarette smoking and raised blood pressure – apply equally to women as to men. In general, however, less favorable CVD rates in men are explained by gender differences in risk factors with smoking and obesity being the major explanatory variables[5]; the gender differences persist whether adjusted for risk factor differences[6] or stratified by level of risk factor[7].

Some comparisons of coronary risk factor associations between men and women are age-dependent. Systolic blood pressure peaks in men at about 60 years but continues to increase in women until about age 80. High density lipoprotein (HDL) cholesterol in women is higher than for men across the life span, particularly in postmenopausal years, and only a modest decline in HDL cholesterol is associated with menopause. Even so, women in the highest quintile of cholesterol (> 7.2 mmol/l) still have lower CHD rates than men in the lowest male quintile (< 5.0 mmol/l) both pre- and postmenopausally[7].

Cigarette smoking, a mass habit of the twentieth century, is a powerful risk factor for CVD in women and in men. Smoking is the most readily modifiable cardiovascular risk factor since it is under the influence of a number of social, cultural and economic influences. There is increasing evidence that regular exposure to passive smoking at home or at work increases the risk of both heart disease and stroke in non-smoking women[8]. Cigarette smoking by women has not yet become widespread in many countries, and there is still time to take global action to protect the health of women by halting the spread of products of the tobacco industry.

Regular physical activity in postmenopausal women is associated with a reduced risk of CVD of one-quarter[9]. Even infrequent moderate activity, as little as once per week, is associated with a reduced risk of death compared with those with sedentary lifestyles. Because a large proportion of the female population is physically inactive and relative risks are of the same magnitude as with other major risk factors, it appears that much CVD can be attributed to physical inactivity.

The relationship of alcohol consumption to CHD is both complex and controversial. The protective effect of alcohol intake at moderate levels is stronger for heart disease than for stroke; the benefit is not sustained at high levels of intake. From a public health perspective, alcohol consumption should continue to be limited; as with all activities directed at individuals, only people at higher absolute risk of heart disease should drink (lightly) for their cardiovascular health[10].

The only risk factors which exert a stronger effect on women than on men are diabetes, low HDL cholesterol and high triglycerides. Diabetes is associated with a 2-fold increased relative risk of CHD in women compared with men[11]. It has been suggested that a better understanding of how diabetes increases cardiovascular risk is central to an understanding of the reasons for the gender gap[12].

Gender differences in CVD mortality and morbidity

The wide gender differences in CVD rates can be partly explained by biology; in the absence of cigarette smoking or diabetes mellitus, CHD in premenopausal women is uncommon[13]. Some of the differences could also be explained by different responses by the health system to women's symptoms. For example, women aged 45–64 years have been shown to have twice as many 'silent' myocardial infarctions as men[14]. Women with CHD symptoms are significantly less likely to be referred to a cardiologist, to be hospitalized, to be given cardiac medications, to receive invasive procedures, or to be referred for echo-cardiographic diagnosis, and less likely to have cardiac disease diagnosed[15]. Doctors are also less likely to make lifestyle recommendations to women.

Despite the higher CHD incidence rates in men, following a myocardial infarction, women appear to have higher in-hospital mortality. These paradoxical findings suggest that women with CHD are treated differently. However, data from community based registers reveal that women have a lower case fatality before admission, and the higher case fatality after an acute event in women admitted to hospital is largely explained by confounding[16,17].

Menopause and coronary heart disease

The age at which menopause occurs is around 50 years and is relatively constant throughout different societies. The only variable which has been shown to affect age at menopause is smoking: smokers reach menopause 1.8 years before non-smokers[18].

Menopause carries a wide variety of cultural and social meanings. In many developing countries, by the time a woman reaches menopause her health may already have been undermined, not by her hormonal state, but by the aftermath of health problems in reproductive years and the social and environmental conditions under which she lives. In developed countries the majority of women are in good health at the time of menopause. Yet it is in these countries that menopause itself is increasingly being depicted as an illness, or estrogen-deficiency 'disease', responsible for an increased risk of many chronic conditions including CHD. This medicalization of a normal life event has resulted in a dramatic increase in sales of post-menopausal hormones, such that Premarin® is now the leading prescription drug in the United States.

The basis for the theory of estrogenic cardioprotectivity and widespread justification for hormone treatment is the widely held notion that the rate of CHD increases steeply after menopause. A sizeable research and pharmaceutical enterprise is traceable to the belief that the increase risk of CVD is causally related to menopausal estrogenic change[15]. However, as shown in Figures 1 and 2, although the CVD mortality rates increase in women dramatically with increasing age (Figure 1), the basic shape of the relationship (log scale) is a straight line for both men and women (Figure 2) suggesting that the increase in CHD in women is more a reflection of age than of menopause *per se*.

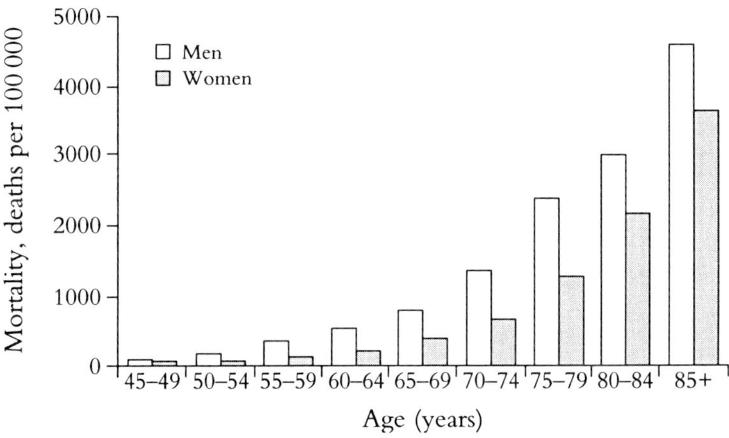

Figure 1   Age-specific coronary heart disease (CHD) mortality per 100 000 population in women and men. New Zealand, 1994

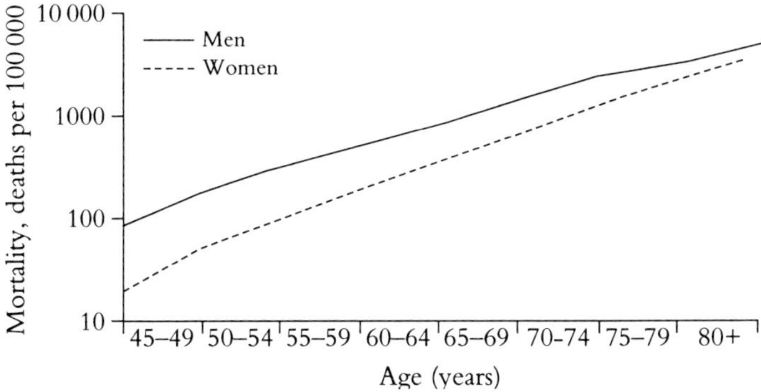

Figure 2   Age-specific coronary heart disease (CHD) mortality per 100 000 population (log scale) in women and men, New Zealand, 1994

Women develop heart disease much later than men and the incidence in women never becomes equal to that in men. The decline in the ratio of male to female deaths that occurs in old age does not reflect an acceleration in women who have been postmenopausal longer, but reflects a slowing of the acceleration that occurs in middle-aged men[12].

The main justification for widespread hormone use arises from the observation from epidemiological studies that estrogen use is associated with a decreased risk of CHD of about one-third[19]. However, data from observational studies are limited by the fact that women who use estrogen have other favorable lifestyle factors that would reduce their risk for heart disease: they smoke less, exercise more, start out with better cholesterol levels, are more closely monitored and are more health conscious[20]. Furthermore, because women who adhere to treatment required (including placebo) have lower mortality risk, it is likely that in any analyses based on current or long-term use of hormone treatment, the benefits would be even further overestimated and the adverse effects underestimated[21].

The data on the effects of prolonged use of postmenopausal hormones and the type of postmenopausal hormones remain limited. The risk of breast cancer (and among women receiving unopposed therapy, the risk of endometrial cancer) rises with increasing duration of treatment, depending on the type of treatment[22]. Current hormone use appears to be associated with a 40% increased risk of breast cancer (relative risk (RR) = 1.40; 95% confidence interval (CI): 1.20–1.63)[23].

Of concern, in a more recent report from the Nurses' Health Study, current (but not past) hormone use was associated with a 35% reduced risk of CVD mortality compared with women who never used hormones[24]. However, in current users who had been taking hormones for 10 years or more, the increase in breast cancer with increased duration of use almost canceled out the favorable association with CHD. The analysis – restricted to unopposed estrogen, a product unsuitable for women with an intact uterus – suggested that combined treatment (estrogen with progestin) did not confer any risks, although the data are confined to only eight cardiac events in 27 161 person-years of follow-up. Most of the benefit in current users was found in women already at high risk; among low-risk women there was no significant benefit.

A meta-analysis of 22 clinical trials involving 4124 women failed to show any statistically significant benefit for hormone users compared with non-users[25]. Again, however, the numbers of CVD events were small, only 12 events in 1818 women in the treatment group and 5 events in 1041 women in the control group. Large randomized controlled trials examining the relationship of hormone treatment to a range of disease outcomes are currently under way, but results will not be available for another decade[26].

In summary, while hormone treatment meets a medical need for women undergoing premature menopause, or for women with severe menopausal symptoms, it is yet to be demonstrated that postmenopausal hormones prevent CVD, or that they are acceptably safe and cost-effective. The recent dramatic increase in the use of hormone treatment for cardio-protection is not supported by the available evidence.

Optimal strategies for prevention

CVD to a large extent is preventable but the two contrasting strategies for primary prevention, the high risk (or individual) strategy and the population (or 'mass') strategy[27], have yet to be optimized. The population strategy aims to reduce the average risk of CVD in the entire community. Since most new cases of CVD occur in people who are at only mildly raised levels of risk, this strategy is likely to have the most impact on reducing the burden of CVD in women.

Most of the interventions which have been demonstrated to impact significantly on CVD can be applied at the population level, for example smoking cessation, dietary changes and physical activity to reduce cholesterol and blood pressure levels and body weight. A healthy cost-effective reduction in the use of tobacco has been achieved in many countries through a population strategy based on strong legislative, fiscal and educational programs; in countries without comprehensive policies, the prevalence of smoking is increasing[5]. Important relationships between risk factor changes in populations and changes in CHD mortality have been demonstrated. For example, in Finland, two-thirds of the decline in mortality from CHD in women between 1970 and 1992 could be explained by changes in the population levels of the three main CVD risk factors[28]; for stroke, half the observed decline in women could be ascribed to population changes in these risk factors[29].

The high-risk strategy involves identifying and treating individuals at high risk of CVD due to elevated blood pressure or the presence of other risk factors. Clinical practice has traditionally been strongly influenced by the epidemiological evidence that the presence of a particular risk factor may double or triple an individual's risk of CVD, or that a particular treatment reduces CVD risk by one-third or one-half – in relative terms. Relative risk estimates, however, only provide information on the strength of an association. An intervention that reduces the relative risk of CHD in women by one-third or one-half seems attractive, but will in fact help only a few women if most of the population are at low or even average risk[30].

High-risk strategies to be both successful and cost-effective require reorientation with the focus on an assessment of absolute risk, not relative risk. As Table 2 shows, the absolute risk (or the likelihood that an individual woman will have an event over a defined period of time) varies markedly according to age as well as the presence or absence of other risk factors[31]. It is noteworthy that at all age groups and in all risk categories, women have a lower absolute risk than men.

An estimate of the probability of a CVD event within the next 8 or 10 years provides a useful approach both for clinicians who wish to convey useful information to patients, and for the development of treatment guidelines. Evidence-based guidelines for treatment of elevated blood pressure and hypercholesterolemia suggest that highest priority for treatment should be given to patients at high absolute risk of one CVD event: older patients, men, and those with multiple risk factors and pre-existing disease[5]. Because the absolute risk of CHD in women remains low until the seventh or eighth decade, any reduction in risk cannot yield great absolute benefits[30].

Table 2 Probability (%) of a cardiovascular disease (CVD) event in women within 8 years, by age and risk factor status. Data from reference[31]

	*Low risk**		*Average risk*		*High risk***	
Age (years)	*Women*	*Men*	*Women*	*Men*	*Women*	*Men*
40	0.7	1.2	1.2	4.1	28.4	70.8
50	2.2	3.7	4.8	11.5	47.0	81.0
60	5.1	7.4	11.9	19.3	60.6	81.7
70	9.0	10.0	19.9	22.9	67.5	84.8

*Low risk: systolic blood pressure (SBP) 105 mmHg, serum cholesterol 185 mg/100 ml, non-smoking, no glucose intolerence, no left ventricular hypertrophy by electrocardiography; **High risk: SBP 185 mmHg, serum cholesterol 335 mg/100 ml, cigarette smoker, glucose intolerance, left ventricular hypertrophy by electrocardiography

An evidence-based approach also has the advantage of allowing an estimate of the number of women at a given level of risk requiring treatment to prevent a CVD event. The number needing treatment (NNT) according to the 5 year probability of developing a CVD event depends on the pre-treatment absolute risk after taking into account all major risk factors (Table 3) and (Figure 3)[32].

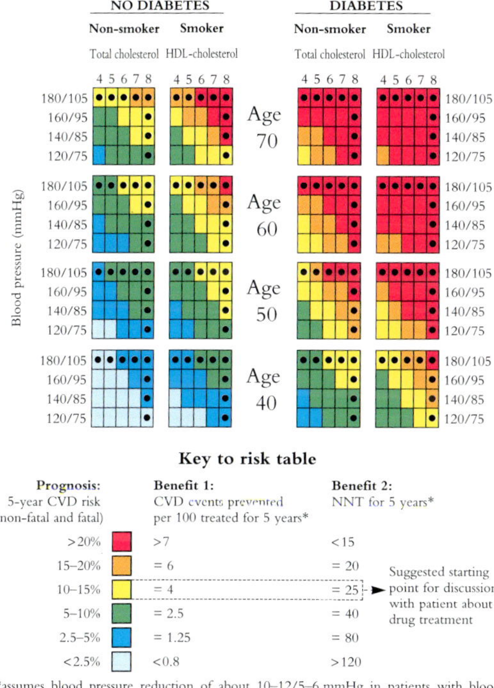

*assumes blood pressure reduction of about 10–12/5–6 mmHg in patients with blood pressure > 140–150/90, or cholesterol reduction of about 20% in patients with total cholesterol >5.0–5.5 mmol/l, produces an approximate 1/3 reduction in CVD risk, whatever the pretreatment absolute risk.

• cells with this marker indicate that in patients with very high levels of cholesterol (>approximately 8.5–9 mmol/l) or blood pressure (>approximately 170–180/100–105 mmHg), the risk equations may underestimate the true risk. **Therefore it is recommended that treatment be considered at lower absolute CVD risk levels than in other patients.**

Table adapted from Recommendations for the Prevention of Coronary Heart Disease in Clinical Practice from the European Societies of Cardiology, Atherosclerosis, and Hypertension.

Figure 3 Benefit of treatment (cardiovascular disease (CVD) events prevented per 100 women treated for 5 years and number needed to treat (NNT) for 5 years) by 5-year absolute risk of a fatal or non-fatal CVD event. This figure can be downloaded in color or black and white from the Oxford Centre for Evidence-Based Medicine, site: http://cebm.jr2.ox.ac.uk/docs/prognosis.html

Table 3 The relation between 5-year cardiovascular disease (CVD) risk and benefit for women: CVD events prevented per 100 patients treated for 5 years, and number needing treatment (NNT) for 5 years to prevent one event

Prognosis: 5-year CVD risk (%) (non-fatal and fatal)	*Benefit 1: CVD events prevented per 100 treated for 5 years*	*Benefit 2: Number needing treatment (NNT) for 5 years*
> 20%	> 7 per 100	< 15
15–20%	6 per 100	20
10–15%	4 per 100	25
5–10%	2.5 per 100	40
2.5–5%	1.25 per 100	80
< 2.5%	< 0.8 per 100	> 120

An evidence-based approach to treatment decisions concerning the use of hormone treatment for cardio-protection based on absolute risk is warranted. The current evidence suggests that the women who would gain the most from treatment would be those at low risk of breast cancer and at high absolute risk of CVD, that is, women who smoke, have high blood pressure, high cholesterol and are obese. Since a woman with a history of CVD is already at a substantial risk of another event (and decreased life expectancy), it is possible that such women, especially if at low risk of breast cancer, would stand to gain most from hormone treatment (Table 4)[22]. On the other hand, many non-pharmacological steps are available to individual women to reduce these risks. Although the two primary prevention strategies are complementary, the population approach has greater potential than the individual high-risk approach and is necessary wherever risk is widely diffused throughout the population. By definition, the individual, or high-risk strategy is limited – and costly – and does not offer a realistic solution to the CVD epidemic, especially in developing countries. A framework for CVD risk-reduction strategies is shown in Table 5.

Present challenges and future prospects

In summary, CVD is the leading cause of death in adult women, and disability associated with CVD in women is projected to become more important in all regions of the world in future decades. Women share with men the same CVD risk factors. There is evidence that lifestyle changes (smoking cessation, adopting healthy eating patterns, engaging in moderate

Table 4 Impact of long-term hormone treatment on life expectancy at age 50 by risk factor status. Data from reference 22 with permission

	Life expectant (years)	*Net change in life expectancy* (years)	
	No treatment	*Estrogen*	*Estrogen + progestin*
No risk factors	82.8	+0.9	+0.1
With hysterectomy	82.8	+1.1	–
At risk of hip fracture	82.4	+1.0	+0.2
At risk of breast cancer	82.3	+0.7	−0.5
At risk of CHD	79.6	+1.5	+0.6
With CHD	76.0	+2.1	+0.9

CHD, coronary heart disease

physical activity and controlling weight) are beneficial for reducing CVD and improving overall health in women as well as men. The strategies for cardiovascular disease prevention for women are similar to those available for men. There is a need for a reappraisal of the widespread use of hormones for cardio-protectivity given the unfavorable risk–benefit trade-off in all but selected groups of women.

While many risk factors are associated with heart disease and stroke, applying our knowledge to effecting change in just three key risk factors is the most immediate challenge. The critical task now, after almost half a century of epidemiological research on cardiovascular disease, is to translate the accumulated evidence into successful primary prevention. Progress has been disappointingly slow. Effective prevention in the long term requires recognition that there are many influences on individual risk and that socio-economic factors also operate through the standard risk factors.

More effort will need to be directed in the future to the social and economic determinants of heart disease and stroke and their interactions with modifiable risk factors. Current approaches directed at high-risk individuals can be optimized by the development of evidence-based treatment guidelines based on absolute risks and benefits. The development of such guidelines should involve the participation of women consumers, as such an approach may superficially appear to disadvantage women. Because women are at lower risk for CVD than men, inevitably, age for age, more men will be treated than women.

Global aging is the main driving force of the CVD epidemic but the risk factor profiles of many populations are changing in an adverse direction.

Table 5 Cardiovascular disease risk reduction objectives and strategies for women

Risk factor	Population strategy (whole population)	Population strategy (directed at women)	High risk strategy at individual women
Hypertension	Inter-sectoral collaboration with food manufacturers, industry, advertisers; eg salt reduction in manufactured food; promotion of a heart–healthy diet	Promotion of relevant and realistic physical activity/movement programs; promote low intake of alcohol in older women	Lifestyle advice; to high absolute risk established evidence eg: 10–15% risk if a CVD event over en-suing 5 years as a starting point for discussion concerning treatment
Cholesterol	As above; increased physical activity; weight control	As above; as for total population (modified)	Dietary counseling at high absolute risk determined guidelines
Current smoker	Comprehensive policies; tobacco control legislation	As for total population	Subsidized smoking programs
Physically inactive	Information and education; accessible activity programs; discouragement of individualized transport	Promotion of community based exercise programs, eg. walking groups	Counseling by primary care physicians; women's health initiatives
Obesity	Nutrition and exercise programs	As for total population (modified)	Dietary counseling exercise and fitness programs

The population approach requires greater attention. Only this strategy can begin to confront the underlying determinants of the global CVD epidemic. Despite the importance of cardiovascular disease in aging populations, few studies have specifically examined older women; the dearth of data is even greater for developing countries. In the meantime, enough is known to make appreciable gains in the prevention and postponement of heart disease and stroke in both women and men. Turning this epidemiological knowledge into policy and practice is the real challenge and will involve enlightened leadership, healthy public policy, and resources for specific CVD prevention programs which take into account the special needs of women.

REFERENCES

1. *Global Burden of Disease.* Murray, C. J. L., Lopez, A. D. eds. (1997). Harvard School of Public Health: Harvard University Press
2. Murray, C. J. L. and Lopez, A. D. (1997). Mortality by cause for eight regions of the world: study. *Lancet*, **349**, 1269–76
3. WHO MONICA Project. Tunsdall-Pedoe, H., Kuulasmaa, K., Amouyel, P., *et al.* (1994). Myocardial infarction and coronary deaths in the World Health Organisation MONICA Project: registration procedures, event rates and case fatality in 38 populations from 21 countries in four continents. *Circulation*, **90**, 583–612
4. Bonita, R. and Beaglehole, R. (1993). Cerebrovascular disease: explaining stroke mortality trends. *Lancet*, **341**, 1510–11
5. Jackson, R. for the WHO MONICA Project and ARIC Study. Gender differences in ischaemic heart disease mortality and risk factors in 46 communities: an ecologic analysis. *CVD Risk Factors* (in press)
6. Wingard, D. L., Suarez, L. and Barrett-Connor, E. (1983). The sex differential in mortality from all causes and ischemic heart disease. *Am. J. Epidemiol.*, **117**, 165–72
7. Isles, C. G., Hole, D. J., Hawthorne, V. M. *et al.* (1992). Relation between coronary risk and coronary mortality in women in the Renfrew and Paisley survey: comparison with men. *Lancet*, **339**, 702–6
8. Kawachi, I., Colditz, G. A., Speizer, F. E., *et al.* (1997). A prospective study of passive smoking and coronary heart disease. *Circulation*, **95**, 237–9

9. Kushi, L. H., Fee, R. M., Folsom, A. R., *et al.* (1997). Physical activity and mortality in post menopausal women. *J. Am. Med. Assoc.*, **277**, 1287–92

10. Jackson, R., Scragg, R. and Beaglehole, R. (1991). Alcohol consumption and risk of coronary heart disease. *Br. Med. J.*, **303**, 211–16

11. Barrett-Connor, E., Cohn, B. A., Wingard, D. L. *et al.* (1991). Why is diabetes mellitus a stronger risk factor for fatal ischemic heart disease in women than in men? *J. Am. Med. Assoc.*, **265**, 627–31

12. Barrett-Connor, E. (1997). Sex differences in coronary heart disease: why are women so superior? *Circulation*, **95**, 252–64

13. Barrett-Connor, E. (1996). The menopause, hormone replacement, and cardiovascular disease: the epidemiologic evidence. *Maturitas*, **23**, 227–34

14. Cohn, P. F. (1988). Silent myocardial ischaemia. *Ann. Int. Med.* **109**, 312–17

15. McKinlay, J. (1996). Some contributions from the social system to gender inequalities in heart disease. *J. Health Soc. Behav.*, **37**, 1–26

16. Sonke, G. S., Beaglehole, R., Stewart, A. W. *et al.* (1996). Sex differences in case fatality before and after admission to hospital after acute cardiac events: analysis of comunity based CHD register. *Br. Med. J.* **313**, 853–5

17. Tunstall-Pedoe, H., Morrison, C., Woodward, M. *et al.* (1996). Sex differences in myocardial infarction and coronary deaths in Scottish MONICA population of Glasgow 1985 to 1991: presentation, diagnosis, treatment, and 28-day case fatality of 3991 events in men and 1551 events in women. *Circulation*, **93**, 1981–92

18. McKinlay, S., Brambilla, D. J. and Posner, J. (1992). The normal menopause transition. *Am. J. Hum. Biol.*, **4**, 37–46

19. Stampfer, M. J. and Colditz, D. A. (1991). Estrogen replacement therapy and coronary heart disease: a quantitative assessment of the epidemiologic evidence. *Preventive Med.*, **20**, 47–63

20. Egeland, G. M., Pullar, L. H., Matthews, K. A. *et al.* (1991). Premenopausal determinants of menopausal oestrogen use. *Preventive Med.*, **20**, 343–9

21. Horowitz, R. I., Biscoli, C. M., Berkman, L. *et al.* (1990). Treatment adherence and risk of death after a myocardial infarction. *Lancet*, **336**, 542–5

22. Grady, D., Ruben, S. M., Petitti, D. B. *et al.* (1992). Hormone replacement therapy to prevent disease and prolong life in post-menopausal women. *Ann. Int. Med.* **117**, 1016–37

23. Colditz, G. A., Egan, K. and Stampfer, M. J. (1993). Hormone replacement therapy and risk of breast cancer: results from epidemiologic studies. *Obstet. Gynecol.* 1473–80

24. Grodstein, F., Stampfer, N. J., Manson, J. E. *et al.* (1996). Post-menopausal estrogen and progestin use and the risk of cardiovascular disease. *N. Engl. J. Med.*, **335**, 453–61

25. Hemminki, E. and McPherson, K. (1997). Impact of postmenopausal hormone therapy on cardiovascular events and cancer: pooled data from clinical trials. *Br. Med. J.* **315**, 149–53

26. Peterson, E. D. and Califf, R. M. (1995). The complexity of studying coronary heart disease in women. *Ann. Epidemiol*, **5**, 79–81

27. Rose, G. Sick individuals and sick populations. (1985). *Int. J. Epidemiol.*, **14**, 32–8

28. Vartiainen, E., Puska, P., Pekkanen, J. *et al.* (1994). Changes in risk factors explain changes in mortality from ischaemic heart disease in Finland. *Br. Med. J.*, **309**, 23–7

29. Vartiainen, E., Sarti, C., Tuomilehto, J. *et al.* (1995). Do changes in cardiovascular risk factors explain changes in mortality from stroke in Finland? *Br. Med. J.*, **310**, 901–4

30. Newham, H. H. and Silberberg, J. (1997). Women's hearts are hard to break. *Lancet*, **349**, s13–s16

31. Cupples, L. A. and D'Agostino, R. B. (1987). Section 34. Some risk factors related to the annual incidence of cardiovascular disease and death using pooled repeated biennial measurements: Framingham Heart Study, 30-year follow-up. In Kannel, W. B., Wolf, P. A., Garrison, R. J. (eds). *The Framingham Study: An Epidemiological Investigation of Cardiovascular Disease*. Bethesda, MD. National Heart, Lung and Blood Institute publication No. (NIM), 87–2703

32. Guidelines for the management of mild blood pressure (1995). National Health Committee, Ministry of Health, Wellington

5

Non-invasive vascular imaging

C. B. Higgins

INTRODUCTION

Degenerative cardiovascular disease is a major cause of death and morbidity in advanced industrialized countries. For instance, statistics of the American Heart Association for 1995 indicate that approximately 11 200 000 people in the United States have a history of myocardial infarction and/or chronic angina pectoris. This includes 1.5 million new acute myocardial infarctions in 1995 with about a 35 per cent mortality. With a high percentage of the population consisting of elderly subjects in many countries, degenerative cardiovascular disease will continue to be a very important public health problem.

The two major degenerative processes of the cardiovascular system are: atherosclerosis consisting of intimal deposition of lipid cholesterol-containing plaque, and arteriosclerosis, loss of elasticity with thickening and hardening of the arteries. Atherosclerosis causes mortality and morbidity principally by obstructing coronary, carotid and peripheral limb arteries. Arteriosclerosis is responsible for aortic aneurysms and may be a major contributing factor for the increasing incidence of heart failure in the elderly. This process causes reduction in aortic and arterial compliance; reduced arterial compliance is now being indicated in the pathogenesis of dilated cardiomyopathy (heart failure) in the elderly.

Up to the current time, most diagnostic and therapeutic techniques have been focused upon symptomatic disease. However, most of the natural history of diseases consists of a long asymptomatic period, during which the pathological process is frequently reversible, hence therapeutic approaches are most effective in this asymptomatic period.

New non-invasive vascular imaging techniques, which have been introduced or refined in the past decade, can provide precise evaluation of vascular pathoanatomy and pathophysiology. Some of these techniques are effective for screening the population for degenerative cardiovascular diseases. The information to be acquired by imaging techniques is: identification and assessment of the severity of vascular stenoses; estimation of arterial compliance; quantification of flow and flow reserve; and characterization of atherosclerotic plaques and other obstructive lesions. Moreover, a screening method for identifying patients with coronary atherosclerosis and those at high risk for coronary events is essential for reducing mortality and morbidity of cardiovascular disease in the aging population.

NON-INVASIVE IDENTIFICATION OF VASCULAR PATHOANATOMY

Magnetic resonance angiography (MRA) has been recognized for several years to be accurate for the demonstration of stenosis of the carotid and vertebral arteries[1]. Three-dimensional time–of–flight MRA after the injection of contrast medium (gadolinium chelates) has become the preferred method for the evaluation of thoracic and abdominal aortic aneurysms[2,3]. Image quality has been considerably improved with improving technology, which permits acquisition of the three-dimensional MRA during a breath-hold period of about 15 s (Fig. 1). Breath-hold contrast-enhanced MRA is now effective for the identification of renal arterial stenosis and constitutes a non-invasive technique for screening patients with suspected renovascular hypertension[4]. This technique is also attractive for the follow–up of renal arterial morphology after angioplasty.

Contrast-enhanced spiral computed tomography (CT) is also very effective for the evaluation of aortic and renal arterial diseases. Three-dimensional reconstruction of CT data acquired in the axial plane is used to display vascular pathology.

ESTIMATION OF ARTERIAL (AORTIC) COMPLIANCE

Arteriosclerosis is degeneration of the arterial wall due to loss of elastin and increase in collagen. This causes increased stiffness or loss of compliance of the arteries. It usually occurs in association with atherosclerosis. Arterial compliance is decreased in patients with hyperlipedemia, hypertension and diabetes.

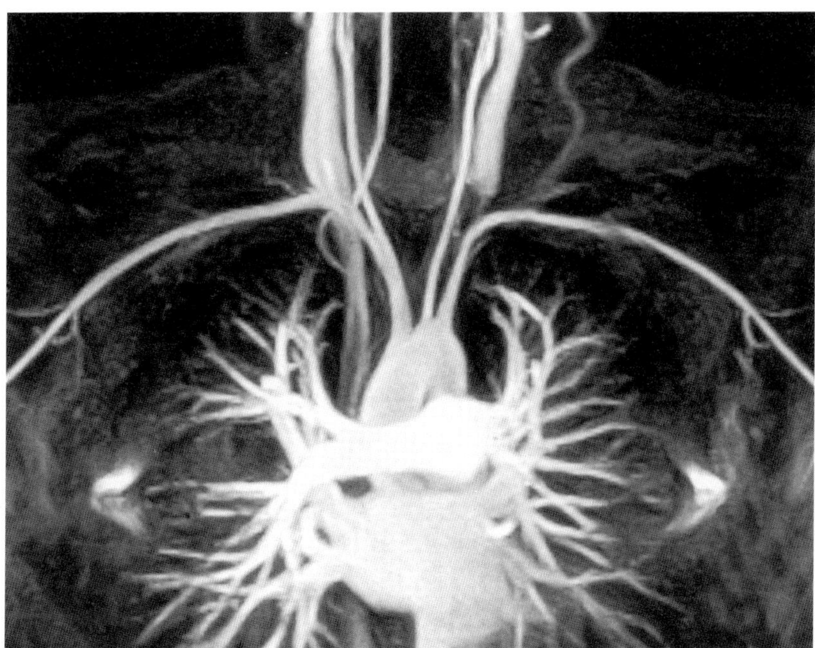

Figure 1 Three-dimensional magnetic resonance angiogram with breath holding during injection of magnetic resonance contrast medium

Compliance is the change in volume of the vessel per change in pressure. A decline in aortic compliance increases the impedance to ventricular ejection and consequently, increases cardiac work and decreases cardiac efficiency. Aortic compliance is a determinant of left ventricular afterload. In patients with reduced ventricular reserve, reduced aortic compliance may contribute to myocardial failure. This factor may be important in the increasing incidence of heart failure in the aging population.

Electrocardiographic-gated magnetic resonance (MR) imaging can be used to measure and monitor aortic compliance[5]. Using images acquired perpendicular to a specified level of the thoracic aorta at end diastole and end systole, the change in volume from end diastole to end systole can be measured. The pulse pressure is measured with a sphygmomanometer. Compliance is measured as the ratio of volume change to pressure change. A decrease in aortic compliance measured by this technique has been observed with advancing decades of age. Aortic compliance has been shown to be higher in athletes and lower in patients with coronary artery disease.

Ventricular ejection produces pressure and flow waves in the aorta. The velocity of pressure and flow waves is determined by compliance of the aortic wall. Aortic flow wave velocity can be measured by velocity-encoded cine MR imaging. Velocity-encoded images perpendicular to the ascending and descending thoracic aorta permit measurement of the time difference between arrival of the flow wave at the imaging site in the ascending and descending aorta. The flow wave velocity has been shown by Mohiaddin *et al.*[5] to increase with age. There is an inverse relationship between flow wave velocity and regional arterial (aortic) compliance.

Thus, MR technique can be used to evaluate the effect of aging on the aorta. Measurements of aortic compliance can be employed to assess the presence and severity of vascular degenerative diseases.

EVALUATION OF CORONARY ANATOMY AND FLOW WITH MR IMAGING

Magnetic resonance angiography (MRA) is a new non-invasive method for displaying coronary arterial anatomy (Figure 2). MRA of the coronary arteries has been shown to be effective for demonstrating coronary arterial stenosis[6–8]. While an early report showed an approximately 90 per cent correlation with coronary X-ray cine angiography for identifying hemo-dynamically significant stenosis[6], subsequently there has been a wide variability among studies regarding diagnostic accuracy[7,8].

Velocity-encoded cine MR imaging has been used to measure blood flow velocity and volume flow in coronary arteries in the basal state and during near maximal coronary vasodilatation induced by dipyridamole (Figure 3)[9]. Using this technique, coronary flow reserve was shown to be diminished in patients with significant stenosis of the left anterior descending coronary artery. Velocity-encoded cine MR imaging of the coronary sinus and measurement of left ventricular mass from cine MR imaging have permitted the assessment of total left ventricular myocardial blood flow expressed as ml/min/g of myocardium. This measurement performed in the basal and vasodilatated state provides evaluation of coronary flow reserve. Abnormal coronary flow reserve has been shown in patients with cardiac transplants, hypertension and hypertrophic cardiomyopathy. Abnormal coronary flow reserve has also been demonstrated in smokers, elderly subjects and postmenopausal women. This technique may prove useful for

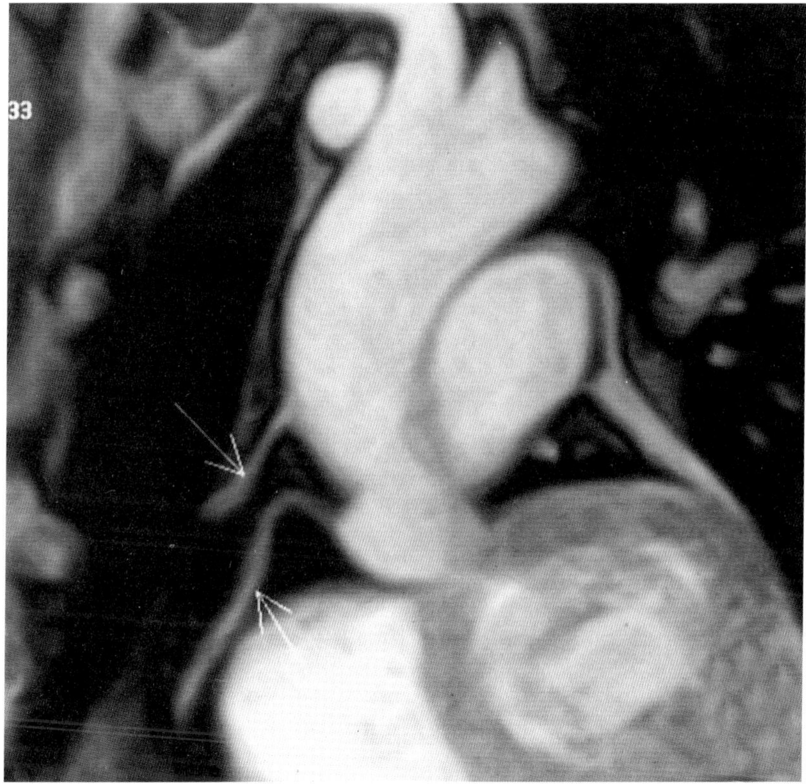

Figure 2 Two-dimensional magnetic resonance angiogram of right coronary artery (arrow) and by pass graft (arrow) during breath hold

verifying the effectiveness of drugs employed to improve coronary vaso-activity.

SCREENING FOR CORONARY ARTERY DISEASE USING ELECTRON BEAM COMPUTED TOMOGRAPHY

Electron beam computed tomography (EBCT) can provide a complete CT scan in as little as 50 ms. EBCT scan without contrast medium is a highly sensitive method for detecting coronary arterial calcification and for quantifying the amount of calcification in the coronary arteries (coronary artery calcification score) (Figure 4). The coronary calcification score increases

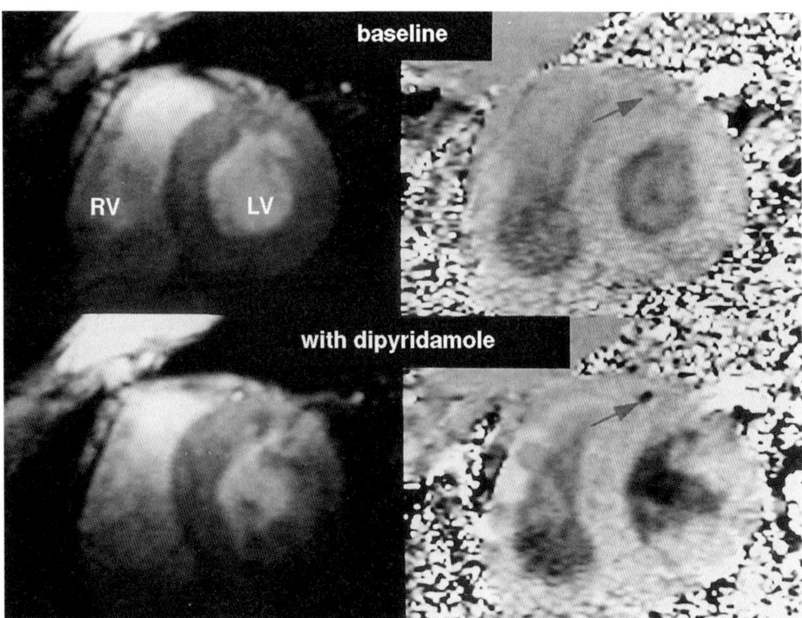

Figure 3 Magnitude and velocity images of heart. Flow velocity is measured in left anterior descending artery (arrows) at baseline and after maximal vasodilatatory effect produced by dipyridamole. RV, right ventricle; LV, left ventricle

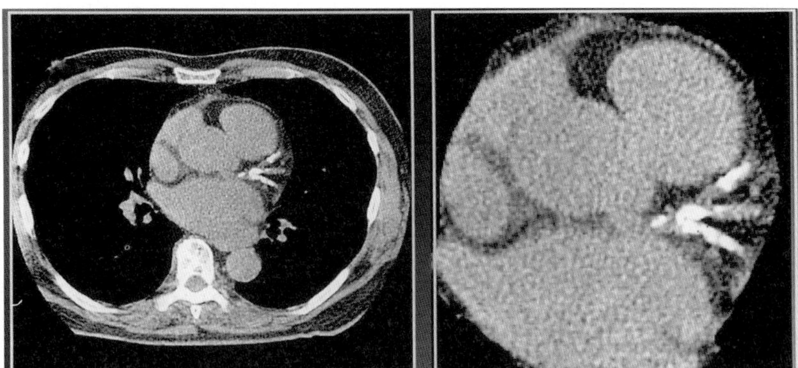

Figure 4 Electron beam computed tomography scan of proximal left coronary artery demonstrated severe coronary calcification

with decades of age, but at any decade the score can discriminate between groups of patients with and without symptomatic coronary arterial disease[10,11]. Kouji *et al.*[12] showed that the coronary artery calcification score had greater diagnostic accuracy for detecting hemodynamically significant coronary artery disease compared to stress electrocardiography and stress thallium testing. In about 1100 asymptomatic patients, this score was significantly associated with new coronary events over a 19-month follow-up period[13].

Contrast-enhanced EBCT angiography of the coronary arteries has been shown to provide excellent depiction of the major coronary arteries (Figure 5)[14,15]. The correlation between EBCT and coronary X-ray angiography has been approximately 80 per cent. A scenario for screening patients for significant coronary arterial disease is to initially use EBCT for quantifying coronary calcification. In those patients with a coronary calcification score

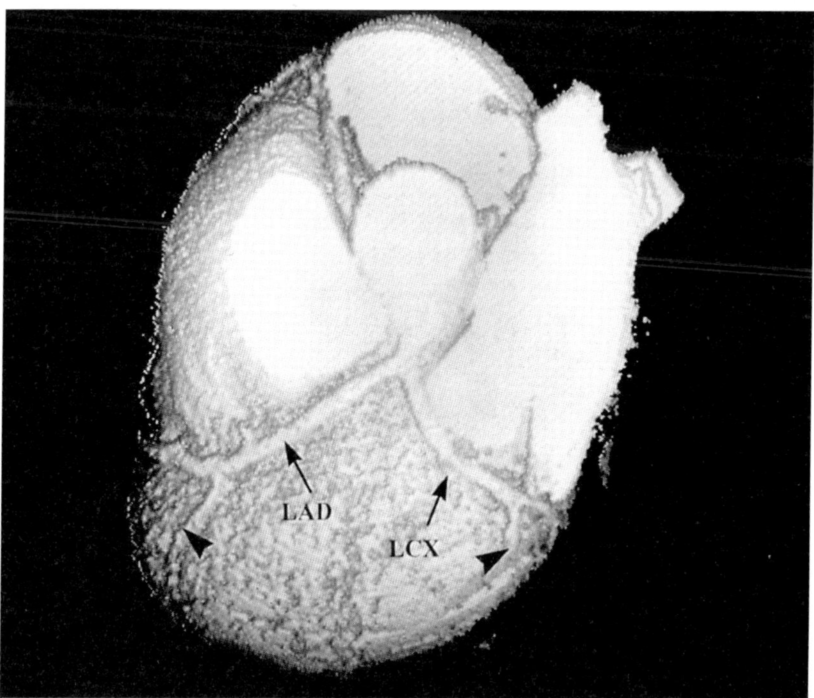

Figure 5 Contrast enhanced electron beam computed tomography scan of coronary arteries with 3D display shows the left anterior descending (LAD) and circumflex (LCX) arteries and major branches (arrowheads)

above a specified threshold for age, EBCT coronary angiography might then be done to identify hemodynamically significant stenosis. Such patients might then undergo coronary catheterization to further evaluate possible critical stenoses and to guide interventional procedures.

CHARACTERIZATION OF ATHEROSCLEROTIC PLAQUE

Intravascular ultrasonography, using a transducer mounted on the tip of a catheter, has been used to depict mural lesions in the coronary arteries. Mural plaque can be identified by intravascular ultrasound in some patients who are considered to have normal coronary arteriogram. This technique has been used to demonstrate the mural injury and improvement in luminal diameter induced by coronary balloon angioplasty. Using analysis of back scattered ultrasound, it has been possible to characterize the material causing obstruction of coronary arteries and the composition of mural plaques.

Intravascular MR imaging has been carried out using a radio frequency coil on the tip of a catheter. With this technique, it has been possible to assess the relative amount of lipid and fibrous tissue in atherosclerotic plaques. This technique has been used to attempt to differentiate between unstable and stable plaques as reflected by the amount of collagenous plaque covering atherosclerotic deposits.

Much further research is necessary before either intravascular ultrasonography or intravascular MR imaging can be used to reliably characterize mural plaque. However, this may prove to be an attractive technique for identifying plaques with a proclivity for rupture and thereby produce thrombotic occlusion.

REFERENCES

1. Anderson, C. M. (1997). MRA of the aortic arch and extracranial carotid arteries. In Higgins C. B., Hricak, H., Helms, C. A., (eds.) *MRI of the Body*, 3rd edn. Philadelphia: Lippincott-Raven, 1369–82
2. Prince, M. R., Narasimham, D. L., Jacoby, W. T., *et al.* (1996). Three-dimensional gadolinium-enhanced MR angiography of the thoracic aorta. *Am. J. Rheumatol.*, **166**, 1387–97

3. Prince, R. P., Narasimham, D. L., Stanley, J. C., *et al.* (1995). Gadolinium-enhanced magnetic resonance angiography of abdominal aortic aneurysms. *J. Vas. Surg.*, Vol. 21, **4**, 656–69

4. Rieumont, M. J., Kaufman, J. A., Geller, S. C., *et al.* (1997). Evaluation of renal artery stenosis with dynamic gadolinium-enhanced MR angiography. *Am. J. Rheumatol.*, **169**, 39–44

5. Mohiaddin, R. H., Underwood, S. R., Bogren, H. G., *et al.* (1989). Regional aortic compliance studied by MRI: the effect of age, training, and coronary artery disease. *Br. Heart J.*, **62**, 90–6

6. Manning, W. J., Wei Li, Edelman, R. R. (1993). A preliminary report comparing magnetic resonance coronary angiography with conventional angiography. *N. Engl. J. Med.*, **328**, 828–32

7. Duerinckx, A. J., Urman, M. K. (1994). Two-dimensional coronary MR angiography: analysis of initial clinical results. *Radiology*, **193**, 731–8

8. Pennell, D. J., Keegan, J., Fircmin, D. N., *et al.* (1993). MRI of coronary arteries; technique and preliminary results. *Br. Heart J.*, **70**, 315–20

9. Sakuma, H., Blake, L. M., Amidon, T. M. *et al.* (1996). Coronary flow reserve: measurement in humans with breath-hold velocity-encoded cine MR imaging. *Radiology*, **198**, 745–50

10. Wong, N. D., Detrano, R. C., Abrahamson, D. *et al.* (1995). Coronary artery screening by electron beam CT: facts, controversy, and future. *Circulation*, **92**, 632–6

11. Agatson, A. S., Janowitz, W. R., Hildner, F. J. *et al.* (1990). Quantification of coronary artery calcium using ultrafast CT. *J. Am. Coll. Cardiol.*, **15**, 827–32

12. Kouji, K., Seki, H., Takehoshi, N. *et al.* (1995). Noninvasive prediction of coronary atherosclerosis by quantification of coronary artery calcification using electron beam computed tomography: comparison with electrocardiographic and thallium exercise stress test results. *J. Am. Coll. Cardiol.*, Nov. 1, Vol. 26, **5**, 1209–22

13. Arad, Y., Spadaro, C. A., Goodman, K. *et al.* (1996). Predictive value of electron beam CT of coronary arteries: 19 month follow-up of 1173 asymptomatic subjects. *Circulation*, **93**, 1951–3

14. Chernoff, D. M., Ritchie, C. J., Higgins, C. B. (1997). Evaluation of electron beam CT coronary angiography in healthy subjects. *Am. J. Rheumatol.*, **169**, 93–9

15. Moshage, W. E., Aschenbach, S., Seese, B. *et al.* (1995). Coronary artery stenosis: three-dimensional imaging with ECG-triggered, contrast enhanced electron beam CT. *Radiology*, **196**, 707–14

6

Preventing coronary heart disease: closing the loop

E. Leitersdorf

PLASMA CHOLESTEROL AND CORONARY HEART DISEASE–EARLY INTERVENTION STUDIES

Large-scale epidemiological studies revealed that in men, the risk of coronary heart disease (CHD) mortality is related to the level of plasma cholesterol. In 361 662 men from the Multiple Risk Factor Intervention Trial, it was found that above the 20th percentile for serum cholesterol (181 mg/dl) CHD risk increased progressively. Above the 85th percentile (253 mg/dl) the relative risk was 3.8[1]. The low density lipoprotein (LDL) fraction has subsequently been found to be one of the most important parameters determining the overall coronary risk. Attempts were made to reduce plasma cholesterol levels using a variety of interventions including lifestyle modification and physical activity, as well as drugs. Several studies have suggested that reduction of plasma LDL cholesterol (LDL-C) concentration leads to a decrease in death by CHD. From 1970–1990 important controversies remained which were related to the effect of treatment on total mortality, and the possibility of excess mortality due to non-cardiovascular causes including cancer, depression, suicide and accidents[2].

THE ANGIOGRAPHIC STUDIES

During the last decade, the hydroxymethylglutaryl coenzyme A (HMG CoA) reductase inhibitors (lovastatin, simvastatin, pravastatin, fluvastatin and atorvastatin) have been introduced, a new class of hypolipidemic drugs which have unique pharmacological characteristics. These potent drugs have a profound influence on plasma lipid and lipoprotein concentrations, mainly by the reduction of plasma LDL-C. Several important angiographic

101

studies ('coronary regression trials') have been completed and the results demonstrated that substantial reduction of plasma LDL-C levels is associated with a decrease in the rate of progression and to a lesser extent, in regression, of the coronary arteriosclerotic process[3]. Although in each one of these studies, only a few hundred patients were included, meta-analyses demonstrated an overall favorable effect on clinical endpoints including CHD events[4].

THE CLINICAL ENDPOINT STUDIES

During the last three years the results of three major intervention studies, involving thousands of patients, have been reported. These studies, the 4S[5], WOSCOPS[6] and CARE[7] studies, revealed that treatment with HMG CoA reductase inhibitors for high risk primary prevention, as well as for secondary prevention, is associated with marked reduction in the prevalence of most of the clinical endpoints examined. These studies demonstrated beyond a reasonable doubt that reduction of plasma LDL-C levels is related to a marked reduction in CHD endpoints. The 4S study, which was a secondary prevention trial on patients with high plasma cholesterol levels, also revealed a highly significant decrease in overall death[5]. In the 4S study, reduction in the risk of major coronary events (non-fatal MI and coronary death) was similar for patients in the four quartiles of baseline plasma cholesterol[8]. In the CARE study the risk reduction was similar to that of the 4S except for patients with low baseline LDL-C levels (< 125 mg/dl) who did not benefit from further cholesterol reduction[7]. Therefore, it may now be concluded that the loop is closed, i.e. cholesterol reduction is associated with a decrease in CHD death.

LIPID REDUCTION AND RESTENOSIS OF CORONARY ARTERIES

During the 90th percentile for serum cholesterol there is a gradual and consistent increase in the use of angioplasty and coronary arterial bypass graft (CABG) in CHD patients[9]. Restenosis, post-angioplasty, is a frequent short-term complication of this procedure. It is a distinct pathological process, different from native atherosclerosis[10]. Three short-term studies (Lovastatin Restenosis Trial[11], SHIPS[12] and FLARE[10]) failed to show any impact of HMG CoA reductase inhibitors on restenosis post-angioplasty[13-15]. *Post hoc* analysis of FLARE demonstrated a beneficial effect on the combined clinical endpoint of total mortality and non-fatal myocardial infarction. It remains to be shown whether cholesterol reduction in patients post-transcatheter therapy benefit from long-term administration of HMG CoA reductase inhibitors.

FUTURE DIRECTIONS

Some unresolved questions still remain. Subgroups including women, diabetics, smokers, hypertensives, transplanted patients and patients with congestive heart failure may have more pronounced effects or may benefit less from cholesterol reduction. Regarding several of these subgroups, including women and diabetics, some encouraging results were reported from *post hoc* analyses of major studies[13,14]. It is expected that prospective meta-analyses, as well as additional studies targeted at specific populations and endpoints, will help us to understand the relative importance of this type of intervention in coronary prevention[15].

REFERENCES

1. Martin, M. J., Hulley, S. B., Browner, W. S. *et al.* (1986). Serum cholesterol, blood pressure, and mortality: implications from a cohort of 361,662 men. *Lancet*, **2**, (8513), 933–6
2. Cucherat, M. and Boissel, J. -P. (1993). Meta-analysis of results from clinical trials on prevention of coronary heart disease by lipid-lowering interventions. *Clin. Trial and Meta-Analysis*, **28**, 109–29
3. Schell, W. D. and Myers, J. N. (1997). Regression of atherosclerosis: a review. *Prog. Cardiovasc. Dis.*, **39**, 483–96
4. Rossouw, J. E. (1995). Lipid-lowering interventions in angiographic trials. *Am. J. Cardiol.*, **76**, 86C–92C
5. The Scandinavian Simvastatin Survival Study Group. (1994). Randomized study of cholesterol lowering in 4444 patients with coronary heart disease: the Scandinavian Simvastatin Survival Study (4S). *Lancet*, **344**, 1383–9
6. Sacks, F. M., Pfeffer, M. A., Moye, L. A., *et al.* (1996). The effect of pravastatin on coronary events after myocardial infarction in patients with average cholesterol levels. *N. Engl. J. Med.*, **335**, 1001–9

7. Shepherd, J., Cobbe, S. M., Ford, I., *et al.* (1995). Prevention of coronary heart disease with pravastatin in men with hypercholesterolemia. *N. Engl. J. Med.*, **333**, 1301–7

8. Scandinavian Simvastatin Survival Study Group. (1995). Baseline serum cholesterol and treatment effect in the Scandinavian Simvastatin Survival Study (4S). *Lancet*, **345**, 1274–5

9. Bittl, J. A. (1996). Advances in coronary angioplasty. *N. Engl. J. Med.*, **335**, 1290–302

10. Serruys, P. W. (1997). Presented at the 46th Scientific Session of the American College of Cardiology (ACC) March 16–19, (Anaheim, CA, USA)

11. Weintraub, W. S., Boccuzzi, S. J., Klein, L., *et al.* and the Lovastatin Restenosis Trial study Group. (1994). Lack of effect of lovastatin on restenosis after coronary angioplasty. *N. Engl. J. Med.*, **331**, 1331–7

12. Nakamura, Y., Yamaoka, O., Uchida, K., *et al.* and the SHIga pravastatin study (SHIPS) group. (1996). Pravastatin reduces restenosis after coronary angioplasty of high grade stenotic lesions: results of SHIPS (SHIga Pravastatin Study). *Cardiovasc. Drugs Ther.*, **10**, 475–83

13. Lewis, S. L., Mitchell, J. S., East, C., *et al.* (1996). Women in CARE have earlier and greater response to pravastatin post myocardial infarction. *Circulation*, **94**, (S1):69

14. Pyörälä, K., Pedersen, T. R., Kjekshus, J, *et al.* (1997). Cholesterol lowering with simvastatin improves prognosis of diabetic patients with coronary heart disease. A subgroup analysis of the Scandinavian Simvastatin Survival Study (4S). *Diabetes Care*, **20**, 614–20

15. Simes, R. J. On behalf of the PPP and CTT investigators. (1995). Prospective meta-analysis of cholesterol-lowering studies: the prospective pravastatin pooling (PPP) project and the cholesterol treatment trialists (CTT) collaboration. *Am. J. Cardiol*, **76**, 122C–6C

7

To treat or not to treat dyslipidemia in the asymptomatic elderly

G. R. Thompson

INTRODUCTION

Dyslipidemia is a risk factor for coronary heart disease but the association weakens with increasing age. Despite the lack of evidence of benefit from lipid-lowering therapy in asymptomatic persons over the age of 65, several national and international organizations have issued guidelines advocating the primary prevention of coronary heart disease in the elderly. Some use estimates of absolute risk as the criterion for lipid–lowering intervention. However, sole reliance upon absolute risk may promote the postponement of timely death from coronary heart disease in the elderly at the expense of the prevention of premature death of younger individuals. Taking relative risk into consideration may help overcome this problem.

The answer to the question of whether to treat dyslipidemia in asymptomatic individuals over the age of 65 could have profound consequences for both health and wealth. As illustrated in Figure 1, coronary heart disease (CHD), which is the major consequence of untreated dyslipidemia, was responsible for more than a quarter of all deaths in males in England and Wales in 1995, and for a fifth of all deaths in females. It is apparent that a substantial proportion of deaths from CHD occurred between the ages of 65 and 74 years (31 per cent in males, 20 per cent in females) although the majority occurred after the age of 75 years (48.5 per cent in males and 74 per cent in females). Thus any decision to undertake primary prevention of CHD after the age of 65 would, if successful, have major implications for the demography of death and for health economics. This being so it is imperative that such a decision should only be taken if it is based on firm evidence suggestive of a beneficial and cost-effective outcome.

105

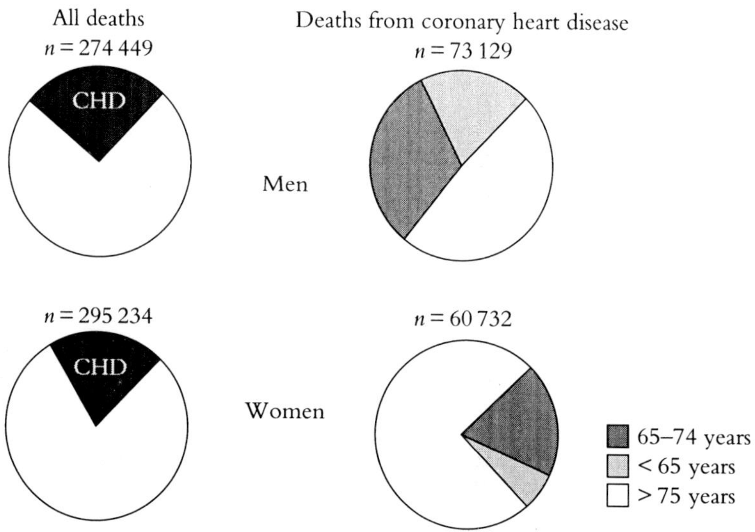

Figure 1 Deaths in England and Wales during 1995 (data from Office for National Statistics, Series DH2, no. 22, London: The Stationery Office)

ROLE OF DYSLIPIDEMIA AS A RISK FACTOR IN THE ELDERLY

Serum cholesterol

Early, albeit indirect, evidence that serum cholesterol is a risk factor for CHD came from Keys *et al.*[1] who showed that serum cholesterol levels fell with increasing age (Figure 2). They interpreted this finding as reflecting better survival of those with lower cholesterol levels, the implication being that high serum cholesterol was a risk factor for premature death.

Direct evidence of a correlation between serum cholesterol and CHD in the elderly has come from the Kaiser Permanente Study which showed that the relative risk for death from CHD in men aged 60–79 years was 1.5 in those in the upper quartile of serum cholesterol compared with the remainder[2]. Analogous results were observed in the Honolulu Heart Study[3] showing that serum total cholesterol remained a risk factor for CHD after the age of 65, despite assertions to the contrary from Framingham.

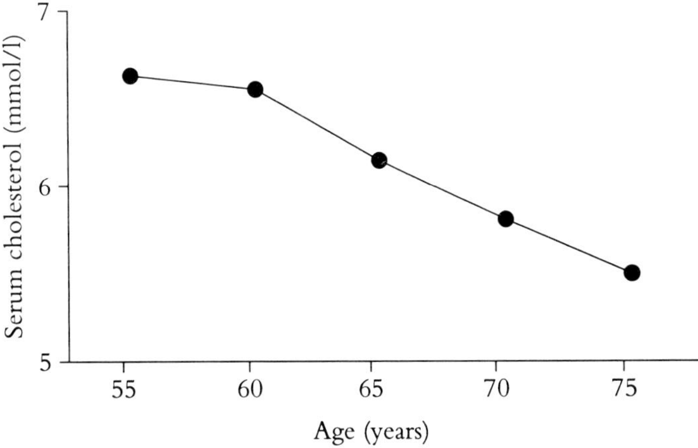

Figure 2 Decrease in serum cholesterol in men with increasing age (data from Keys *et al.*, reference 1)

Further evidence has come from a pooled analysis of 22 studies[4]. Relative risk of death from CHD was significantly higher in those aged ≥ 65 years with serum cholesterol ≥ 6.2 mmol/l compared with < 5.2 mmol/l but the relative risks associated with a raised cholesterol level were much lower than those observed in individuals < 65 years old (men 1.32 versus 1.73 and women 1.12 versus 2.44). A decreasing gradient of relative risk with increasing age has also been observed in subjects with familial hyper-cholesterolemia[5] which implies the existence of varying degrees of suscep-tibility to hypercholesterolemia caused by a raised low-density lipoprotein (LDL) concentration (the 'Churchill' phenomenon).

Recent data from the New Haven Cohort of the Established Population for the Epidemiological Study of the Elderly (EPESE), however, showed no correlation between serum cholesterol and either fatal or non-fatal CHD nor total mortality[6]. A subsequent analysis of all the cohorts participating in EPESE showed that a raised cholesterol level was associated with increased risk of death from CHD but only after adjusting for lower serum iron and albumin, both markers of ill-health, and excluding the CHD deaths which occurred during the first year of follow-up[7]. In this study the trend towards increases in relative risk with increasing cholesterol observed in subjects aged 71–80 years was no longer evident after the age of 80 (Figure 3).

High-density lipoprotein cholesterol and serum triglyceride

An inverse correlation between high-density lipoprotein (HDL) cholesterol and CHD was observed in the Framingham Study[8] and confirmed in EPESE[9]. Again, as with total cholesterol, the relationship was much weaker after the age of 80 (Figure 4). However, another study carried out in men aged 80 and women aged 82 showed that both total and HDL cholesterol remained predictive for new CHD events even at that advanced age[10].

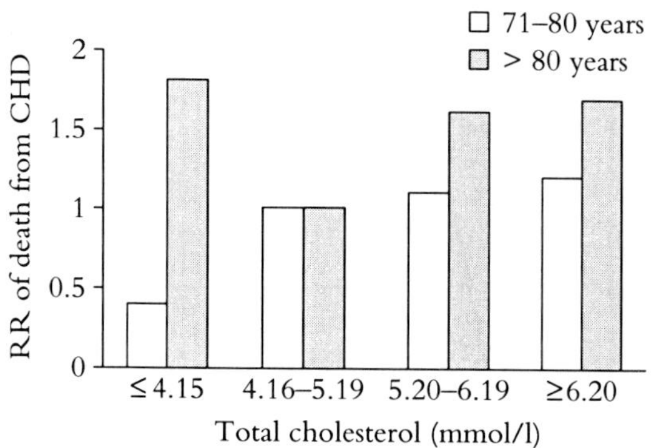

Figure 3 Adjusted relative risk (RR) of fatal CHD according to total cholesterol in 3904 subjects in EPESE (data from Corti *et al.*, reference 9)

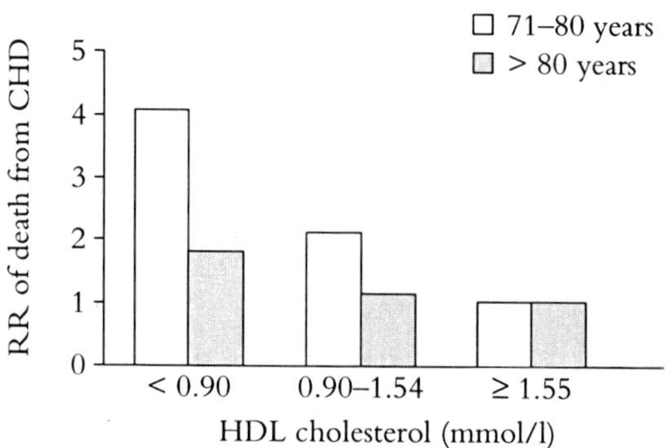

Figure 4 Adjusted relative risk (RR) of fatal CHD according to HDL cholesterol in 3904 subjects in EPESE (data from Corti *et al.*, reference 9)

In a study of 67-year-old Swedish men HDL cholesterol was not measured but fasting serum triglycerides were found to correlate strongly with risk of CHD[11]. An analogous finding emerged from the Physicians' Health Study of men aged 40–84 years in whom non-fasting triglyceride was an independent risk factor for CHD[12]. In contrast triglyceride was not a risk factor in the cohort of eighty-year-olds alluded to previously[10].

EVIDENCE OF BENEFIT FROM LIPID-LOWERING INTERVENTION

The relationship between serum lipid and lipoprotein abnormalities and the risk of developing CHD among the elderly has been reviewed recently in an unbiased and balanced manner[13]. In particular the authors draw attention to the lack of evidence that lipid-lowering therapy is beneficial in the primary prevention of CHD in men and women over the age of 65; this was the upper limit for entry into the West of Scotland Coronary Prevention Study (WOSCOPS), the only large-scale primary prevention trial to have taken place in the current statin era.

The only data which have any bearing on this issue are derived from observational studies which examined changes in risk of CHD associated with decreasing levels of serum cholesterol. The eighteen years follow-up of the Whitehall Study showed that the relative risk of death from CHD was increased less in men aged 65–79 years for each 2 mmol/l increment in serum cholesterol than was the relative risk for men aged 50–64 years[14]. Similarly, in the meta-analysis of Law *et al.*[15], the percentage decrease in CHD mortality associated with each 10 per cent (0.6 mmol/l) decrease in serum cholesterol lessened with increasing age. There is an obvious need for a primary prevention trial of lipid-lowering therapy in subjects over the age of 65 years, with CHD and total mortality as end-points.

LIPID-LOWERING THERAPY FOR PRIMARY PREVENTION OF CHD IN THE ELDERLY: CURRENT ATTITUDES AND GUIDELINES

The case for intervention has been argued cogently by Bilheimer[16] in a detailed review, who draws a distinction between chronological and biological age and advocates basing treatment decisions on the latter criterion.

Although the relative risk of CHD decreases with age, absolute risk rises, which offers considerable scope for lipid–lowering therapy to decrease events. However, the beneficial effects of the latter in the asymptomatic elderly remain hypothetical, apart from the extrapolation of the results of secondary prevention trials such as the Scandinavian Simvastatin Survival Study (4S) and the Cholesterol and Recurrent Events study (CARE), both of which included older subjects than did WOSCOPS.

The opposite viewpoint was taken in two editorials, both of which discouraged treating hypercholesterolemia in the elderly until further evidence becomes available that the benefits outweigh the risks[17,18]. The feasibility of achieving a significant reduction in LDL cholesterol in men and women over the age of 65 has been demonstrated in a pilot study[19] but the trial which was to have followed was canceled through lack of funds. The results of the Anti-hypertensive and Lipid-lowering Treatment to Prevent Heart Attack Trial (ALLHAT), which includes a sub-study of LDL-lowering in 20 000 individuals over the age of 55, will be awaited with great interest[20]. However, this will not be before the year 2002.

Table 1 lists the various national and international organizations which have issued guidelines on lipid-lowering therapy. All concur that age is no bar to secondary prevention of CHD but they differ in their attitudes to primary prevention.

Table 1 Guidelines regarding lipid–lowering therapy for primary prevention of CHD in the hypercholesterolemic but otherwise healthy elderly

Source	*Date*	*Recommendation*
EAS	1992	Treat those ≥ 75 years
BHA	1993	Do not treat > 65 years
NHF (NZ)	1993	Treat those 60–80 years
NCEP II (USA)	1994	No age limit
ESC/EAS/ESH	1994	Treat up to 70 if AR > 2% per annum
Sheffield tables (UK)	1996	Treat up to 70 if AR > 3% per annum
ACP (USA)	1996	Do not screen ≥ 75 years 65–75 years?

AR, Absolute risk of CHD; EAS, European Atherosclerosis Society; BHA, British Hyperlipidaemia Association; NHF (NZ), National Heart Foundation of New Zealand; NCEP II (USA), US National Cholesterol Education Program; ESC/EAS/ESH, European Society of Cardiology/European Atherosclerosis Society/European Society of Hypertension; ACP, American College of Physicians

The European Atherosclerosis Society (EAS) encourages primary prevention up to or even after the age of 75 in asymptomatic individuals with hypercholesterolemia who are otherwise healthy and have a reasonable life expectancy[21]. Similar attitudes were expressed by the National Heart Foundation (NHF) of New Zealand[22] and the US National Cholesterol Education Program (NCEP)[23]. In contrast the British Hyperlipidaemia Association (BHA) does not advocate embarking on lipid-lowering drug therapy after the age of 65[24]. The American College of Physicians (ACP) guidelines for screening (and by implication for treatment) discourage measuring serum cholesterol after the age of 75 and question the benefits of doing so between 65 and 75 years[25]. The joint guidelines of the European Society of Cardiology (ESC), European Atherosclerosis Society (EAS) and European Society of Hypertension (ESH) advocate treating hyperlipidemia up to the age of 70 if the absolute risk of CHD exceeds 20 per cent per 10 years[26]. The same age limit is used by Ramsey *et al.*[27,28] in their Sheffield tables although they stipulate that absolute risk should exceed 30 per cent per 10 years before embarking on lipid-lowering drug therapy.

LIMITATIONS OF ABSOLUTE RISK AS THE SOLE BASIS FOR THERAPEUTIC DECISIONS

As noted above the joint guidelines of the ESC, EAS and ESH and the Sheffield tables both recommend estimating the absolute risk of CHD as a basis for decisions on treatment. In each instance the calculations used are adaptations of the Framingham Risk Score developed by Anderson *et al*[29]. However, both use approximations, the most important of which is eliminating variations in HDL cholesterol from their risk calculations. In view of the importance of HDL cholesterol as a correlate of CHD risk, especially in the elderly as discussed earlier, this modification is liable to introduce major errors in the estimation of risk in individuals with high or low HDL cholesterol levels. The Sheffield tables introduce a second approximation which further limits their validity, namely the fixation of systolic blood pressure so as to render hypertension a dichotomous variable[30].

Both the joint European guidelines and the Sheffield tables include estimates of risk for 70-year-olds, despite the lack of evidence of benefit from lipid-lowering therapy over the age of 65. Accepting that this evidence will eventually be forthcoming, perusal of the corrected set of Sheffield tables[28] indicates that a 70-year-old male smoker with a serum cholesterol of only 5.5 mmol/l is eligible for lipid-lowering drug therapy, despite a relative risk of only 1.8. In contrast the tables specify that serum cholesterol should not even be measured in a normotensive, non-smoking, non-diabetic male without left ventricular hypertrophy until he reaches the age of 64. If, by a 1:500 chance, he happens to have familial hyper-cholesterolemia he may not reach that age if left undiagnosed and untreated.

This leads on to a consideration of the importance of relative risk. This is exemplified by the fact that a 30-year-old non-smoking, non-diabetic male with a systolic blood pressure of 130 mmHg, no left ventricular hypertrophy on ECG and with a serum total cholesterol of 10.4 mmol/l and HDL cholesterol of 1.17 mmol/l has a 10 year risk of a coronary event of only 4.6 per cent but a relative risk of 5.65. On the absolute risk criteria laid down by the three European societies and the Sheffield tables he would not qualify for lipid-lowering therapy. However, if, as is likely with a cholesterol level of > 10 mmol/l at that age, he has familial hyper-cholesterolemia, his relative risk of death from CHD before the age of 39 is known to be increased almost 50-fold (A. Neil, personal communication). Hence both absolute and relative risk need to be taken into account when deciding upon whether to treat.

As a working rule it is suggested that, irrespective of absolute risk, a relative risk of > 4 before the age of 65 merits consideration of treatment of severe hypercholesterolemia. Conversely, individuals above that age would not be eligible for lipid-lowering therapy if their relative risk was < 2, whatever their absolute risk. This should ensure that prevention of premature CHD remains a more important priority than postponing the death, or influencing the cause of death, of septuagenarians and octagenarians.

REFERENCES

1. Keys, A., Mickelsen, O., Miller E. O., *et al.* (1950). The concentration of cholesterol in the blood serum of normal men and its relation to age. *J. Clin. Invest.*, **29**, 1347–53
2. Rubin, S. M., Sidney, S., Black, D. M., *et al.* (1990). High blood cholesterol in elderly men and the excess risk for coronary heart disease. *Ann. Intern. Med.*, **113**, 916–20

3. Benfante, R. and Reed D. (1990). Is elevated serum cholesterol level a risk factor for coronary heart disease in the elderly? *J. Am. Med. Assoc.*, **263**, 393–6

4. Manolio, T. A., Pearson, T. A., Wenger, N. K., *et al.* (1992). Cholesterol and heart disease in older persons and women. Review of an NHLBI Workshop. *Ann. Epidemiol.*, **2**, 161–75

5. Scientific Steering Committee on behalf of the Simon Broome Register Group (1991). Risk of fatal coronary heart disease in familial hypercholesterolaemia. *Br. Med. J.*, **303**, 893–6

6. Krumholz, H. M., Seeman, T. E., Merrill, S. S., *et al.* (1994). Lack of association between cholesterol and coronary heart disease mortality and morbidity and all-cause mortality in persons older than 70. *J. Am. Med. Assoc.*, **272**, 1335–40

7. Corti, M. C., Guaralnik, J. M., Salive, M. E., *et al.* (1997). Clarifying the direct relation between total cholesterol levels and death from coronary heart disease in older persons. *Ann. Intern. Med.*, **126**, 753–60

8. Castelli, W. P., Wilson, P. W., Levy, D., *et al.* (1989). Cardiovascular risk factors in the elderly. *Am. J. Cardiol.*, **63**, 12H–19H

9. Corti, M. C., Guralnik, J. M., Salive, M. E., *et al.* (1995). HDL cholesterol predicts coronary heart disease mortality in older persons. *J. Am. Med. Assoc.*, **274**, 539–44

10. Aronow, W. S., Ahn, C. (1996). Risk factors for new coronary events in a large cohort of very elderly patients with and without coronary artery disease. *Am. J. Cardiol.*, **77**, 864–6

11. Welin, L., Eriksson, H., Larsson, B., *et al.* (1991). Triglycerides, a major coronary risk factor in elderly men. A study of men born in 1913. *Eur. Heart J.*, **12**, 700–4

12. Stampfer, M. J., Krauss, R. M., Ma, J., *et al.* (1996). A prospective study of triglyceride level, low-density lipoprotein particle diameter and risk of myocardial infarction. *J. Am. Med. Assoc.*, **276**, 882–8

13. Corti, M. C., Barbato, G., Baggio, G. (1997). Lipoprotein alterations and atherosclerosis in the elderly. *Curr. Opin. Lipidology,* **8**, 236–41

14. Shipley, M. J., Pocock, S. J., Marmot, M. G. (1991). Does plasma cholesterol concentration predict mortality from coronary heart disease in elderly people? 18 year follow-up in Whitehall study. *Br. Med. J.*, **303**, 89–92

15. Law, M. R., Wald, N. J., Thompson, S. G. (1994). By how much and how quickly does reduction in serum cholesterol concentration lower risk of ischaemic heart disease? *Br. Med. J.*, **308**, 367–72

16. Bilheimer D. W. (1991). Clinical considerations regarding treatment of hyper-cholesterolemia in the elderly. *Atherosclerosis*, **91** (Suppl) S35–57

17. Beaglehole, R. (1991). Coronary heart disease and elderly people. *Br. Med. J.*, **303**, 69–70

18. Hulley, S. B., Newman, T. B. (1994). Cholesterol in the elderly. Is it important? *J. Am. Med. Assoc.*, **272**, 1372–4

19. LaRosa J. C., Applegate, W., Crouse, J. R. III, *et al.* (1994). Cholesterol lowering in the elderly. Results of the Cholesterol Reduction in Seniors Program (CRISP) pilot study. *Arch. Intern. Med.*, **154**, 529–39

20. Davis, B. R., Cutler, J. A., Gordon D. J., *et al.* (1995). Rationale and design for the antihypertensive and lipid lowering treatment to prevent heart attack trial (ALLHAT). *Am. J. Hypertens.*, **9**, 342–60

21. European Atherosclerosis Society International Task Force for Prevention of Coronary Heart Disease (1992). Prevention of coronary heart disease: scientific background and new clinical guidelines. *Nutr Metab Cardiovasc Dis.*, **2**, 113–56

22. Mann J. I., Crooke, M., Fear, H., *et al.* (1993). Guidelines for detection and management of dyslipidaemia. Scientific Committee of the National Heart Foundation of New Zealand. *NZ Med. J.*, **106**, 133–41

23. National Cholesterol Education Program (1994). Second report of the Expert Panel on detection, evaluation and treatment of high blood cholesterol in adults (Adults Treatment Panel II). *Circulation*, **89**, 1329–445

24. Betteridge, D. J., Dodson, P. M., Durrington, P. N., *et al.* (1993). Management of hyperlipidaemia: guidelines of the British Hyperlipidaemia Association. *Postgrad. Med. J.*, **69**, 359–69

25. American College of Physicians (1996). Guidelines for using serum cholesterol, high-density lipoprotein cholesterol, and triglyceride levels as screening tests for preventing coronary heart disease in adults. Clinical guideline, Part 1. *Ann. Intern. Med.*, **124**, 515–17

26. Pyorala, K., De Backer, G., Graham, I., *et al.* (1994). Prevention of coronary heart disease in clinical practice. Recommendations of the Task Force of the European Society of Cardiology, European Atherosclerosis Society and European Society of Hypertension. *Eur. Heart J.*, **15**, 1300–31

27. Ramsay, L. E., Haq, I. U., Jackson, P. R., *et al.* (1996). Targeting lipid lowering drug therapy for primary prevention of coronary heart disease: an updated Sheffield table. *Lancet*, **348**, 387–8

28. Ramsay L. E., Haq, I. U., Jackson, P. R., *et al.* (1996). The Sheffield table for primary prevention of coronary heart disease: corrected. *Lancet*, **348**, 1251–2

29. Anderson, K. M., Wilson, P. W. F., Odell, P. M., *et al.* (1991). An updated coronary risk profile. *Circulation,* **83**, 356–62

30. Haq, I. Q., Jackson, P. R., Yeo, W. W., *et al.* (1995). Sheffield risk and treatment table for cholesterol lowering for primary prevention of coronary heart disease. *Lancet,* **346**, 1467–71

8

HMG CoA reductase inhibitors: cholesterol lowering for all seasons

J. Shepherd

INTRODUCTION

Because of the lack of good evidence based on clinical trials, no-one is really sure how to handle the problem of risk factors in the elderly. If we agree that it is a good thing to lower cholesterol levels in the elderly, however, then the hydroxymethyl glutaryl coenzyme A (HMG CoA) reductase inhibitors are likely to be very effective in doing so. The discovery, development, and marketing of HMG CoA reductase inhibitors over the last 20 years has resolved the major problem of how to lower cholesterol effectively and safely. Independently of patients' age or sex, HMG CoA reductase inhibitors can lower levels of total serum cholesterol (TC) by nearly 30%, low-density lipoprotein (LDL) cholesterol by 35%, and tri-glycerides by more than 25%. In addition they raise serum high–density lipoprotein (HDL) cholesterol by up to 10%[1,2].

HMG CoA REDUCTASE INHIBITORS

Structure and metabolism

As Figure 1 shows, some of these agents (eg simvastatin and lovastatin) are prodrugs that become active when the closed ring structure is opened by lactone hydrolysis *in vivo*. This does not make them any less effective than others, such as pravastatin and fluvastatin, which are already in their active form. HMG CoA reductase inhibitors target the liver, where they are effectively trapped. Very little reaches the systemic circulation, and their half-lives in peripheral blood in general are very short (0.7–2.0 hours) although some agents (particularly atorvastatin) have been engineered to extend their half-life substantially. After oral administration they enter the

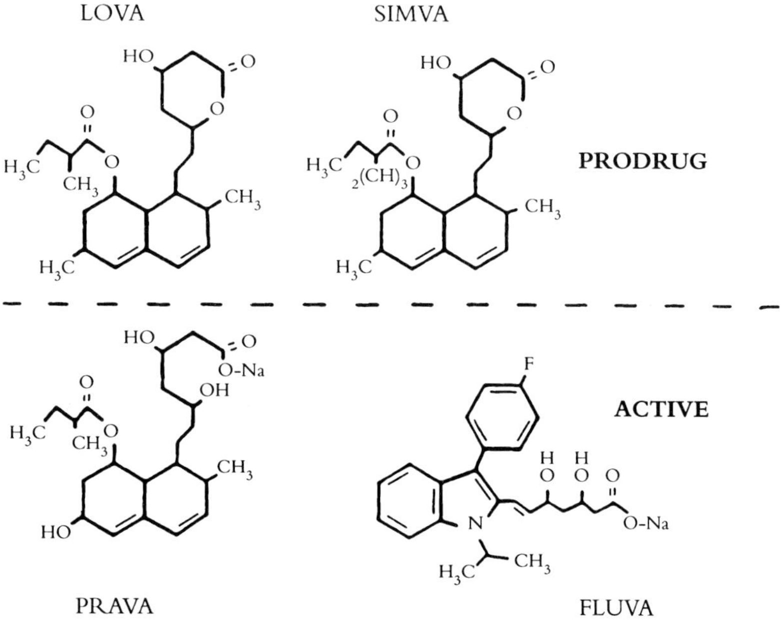

Figure 1 Structural formulae of HMG CoA reductase inhibitors. Lovastatin and simvastatin are prodrugs; pravastatin and fluvastatin are in an active form

liver from the intestine *via* the portal system, the prodrugs being metabolized into the active form on the way. A dose of fluvastatin is almost completely absorbed, while two-thirds of simvastatin and only one-third of lovastatin and pravastatin doses are absorbed. About half of pravastatin and more than 90% of the other HMG CoA reductase inhibitors becomes protein-bound, and they are all excreted largely in the feces.

Mode of action

The active site of HMG CoA reductase inhibitors is the open ring structure mentioned above, which mimics 3-hydroxy-3-methylglutaric acid. It inhibits cholesterol synthesis in the liver by blocking the conversion of 3-hydroxy-3-methylglutarate into mevalonic acid, a major precursor of cholesterol. Deprived of its essential regulatory cholesterol pool, the liver responds by activating specific cell membrane receptors that remove cholesterol-rich lipoproteins from the peripheral blood. So in essence these drugs promote the clearance and breakdown of plasma LDL cholesterol by blocking one hepatic physiological pathway, thereby activating another.

HMG CoA REDUCTASE INHIBITORS IN PRACTICE

HMG CoA reductase inhibitors effectively lower serum cholesterol, and such lowering reduces the risk of cardiovascular disease (CVD). The evidence for this comes from angiographic and event-related studies begun in the late 1980s. The former used angiography or ultrasound evidence of the changes in the atherosclerotic lesions in the arteries of individuals given the drug as a surrogate end-point for event reduction − the real benefit of cholesterol lowering. Event-related studies have investigated the efficacy of these drugs in reducing morbidity and mortality from CVD.

Angiographic studies

Major angiographic studies have included ACAPS[3], CCAIT[4], MARS[5], KAPS[6], PLAC I[7] & II[8], REGRESS[9] and MAAS[10]. Among more recent studies, FLARE has produced results very similar to those of the eight studies just mentioned. These studies used coronary angiography or carotid ultrasound, and involved 151–919 individuals (men only in KAPS and RE-GRESS) treated for 2–4 years with HMG CoA reductase inhibitors or placebo. As Dr Leitersdorf describes elsewhere (pages 101–4) the results were disappointing in one sense and extraordinarily successful in another. Even after up to four years, cholesterol lowering treatment produced little regression of lesions in any of the studies, though it did halt their progression.

However, though these studies were not designed to detect reductions in events related to CVD, meta-analysis of all the results revealed a clear tendency for the patients who received active treatment to have fewer cardiovascular deaths, non-fatal myocardial infarctions (MI), strokes, CABG (coronary artery bypass grafting) and other events than those given placebo; the figures for total events were 167 vs. 261. In fact the larger studies showed significant results in their own right; the figures were 5 vs. 14 for ACAPS (lovastatin; $n = 919$) and 59 vs. 93 for REGRESS (pravastatin; $n = 889$, $p = 0.002$).

So lowering cholesterol produces marginal small angiographic or ultrasound changes in lesions, while having a major impact on events in the lives of those receiving treatment.

Event-related studies

Three major event-related trials have already been published: the West of Scotland Coronary Prevention Study (WOSCOPS), a primary prevention trial using pravastatin and involving 6595 men[2]; the Scandinavian Simvastatin Survival Study (4S) on 4444 subjects[11]; and the Cholesterol And Recent Events (CARE) study, involving 4159 individuals[12]. CARE and 4S were secondary prevention trials, using patients who had previously had a myocardial infarction (MI).

All three trials demonstrated a substantial reduction in cardiovascular events (deaths and nonfatal MIs) over the course of about 5 years. The reductions were 24% in CARE, 31% in WOSCOPS, and 34% in 4S. Most interestingly, these benefits first appeared much earlier than expected (eg after about 6 months of treatment, rather than 2 years, in WOSCOPS). How do HMG CoA reductase inhibitors give such early benefit? They may well have benefit which goes beyond their cholesterol-reducing effect, and this issue is now the subject of intensive laboratory-based clinical investigation. It has been suggested that HMG CoA reductase inhibitors may reduce the frequency of events through an anti-inflammatory effect, by normalizing the arterial endothelium, stabilizing atherosclerotic plaques, and inhibiting lipoprotein oxidation or the formation of platelet-rich thrombi[13].

Whatever the mechanism of an early benefit, it would be particularly important for the elderly, who may not have many years left to wait for any treatment to work.

HMG CoA REDUCTASE INHIBITION AND THE ELDERLY

Some key questions in relation to the utility of HMG CoA reductase inhibitors in the elderly are as follows.

1   Does age alter the relevance of CVD risk factors?

2   Does risk factor reduction work in the elderly?

3   Is cholesterol a risk factor for coronary heart disease in the elderly?

4   Does lipid lowering benefit the elderly in practice?

If elderly people show the same risk factors as those who are middle-aged, and if these risk factors are clearly linked to CVD, will modifying the risk factors make any difference to the presentation of CVD?

Does age alter the relevance of CVD risk factors?

Serum cholesterol levels increase slowly up to 50 years in both sexes, though they are lower in women; thereafter levels tend to reach a plateau or decline in men, while increasing in women after the menopause. So, does the total cholesterol burden over time influence the overall risk of death from CVD?

As Figure 2 shows, relatively more males than females die early from coronary heart disease (CHD)[14], women apparently being protected by their estrogen status. But the relative incidence of such deaths in men tends to stabilize, or even fall, as their cholesterol level stabilizes and falls, while in women it tends to rise progressively, suggesting that the total cholesterol burden over time might actually predict CVD in an individual.

It must be remembered, however, that cholesterol level alone is a poor predictor of CVD, even in middle-aged individuals, and a substantial proportion of people suffering an MI have 'normal' cholesterol levels. In

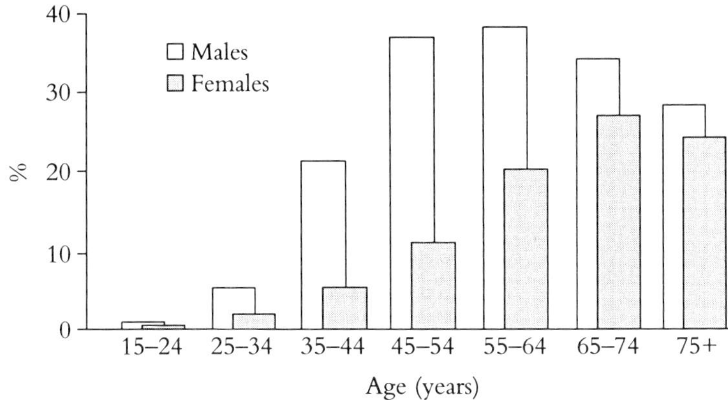

Figure 2   Deaths from coronary heart disease in the USA[14] according to age and sex

addition, the difference in cholesterol level between those who have had an MI and those who have not is about 0.5 mmol/litre in people of 40–45 years, but declines to only 0.1 mmol/litre in 70-year-olds. So cholesterol level is a relatively good predictor in the young and a relatively poor predictor in the elderly; nevertheless, cholesterol is still a significant predictor in elderly people. An individual in the highest quartile of cholesterol in the 75-year age group still has a much higher risk of a myocardial infarction than if he were in the lowest quartile. Although the difference in cholesterol at age 70 years between those who have an MI and those who do not is small, those with high cholesterol are much more likely to have an MI than those with low cholesterol (Figure 3).

Does risk factor reduction work in the elderly?

Some years ago Khaw & Rose reported on a survey in England and Wales of cholesterol levels in individuals[15]. They said that those in whom a cholesterol level greater than 6.5 mmol/litre was reduced by a standard amount were predicted to have reduced their absolute risk much less if they were 35–44 years old than if they were 55–64 years old. This meant that 862 35–44-year-old males (or 4649 women) had to be treated to avoid one event at that age range, whereas at age 55–64 only 104 (or 315) had to be treated to avoid one event. Because the absolute risk of events is far greater in the higher than in the lower age range, the number of events prevented is far greater if the older rather than younger individuals are treated (for example 11 568 vs. 1371 events prevented in treated males of 55–64 and 35–44 years respectively)[15]. However, the relative risk is also important here; treating all the elderly in our population would leave no resources for the middle-aged who may well have a much longer future ahead of them.

Is cholesterol a risk factor for coronary heart disease in the elderly?

Alongside this question one must consider risk indicated by individuals' co-morbidity and frailty, as indices of debility. The three-center US Epidemiological Study of the Elderly (EPESE) was set up in 1988[17]. The mean age of the 4066 male and female participants was 79.2 years at baseline.

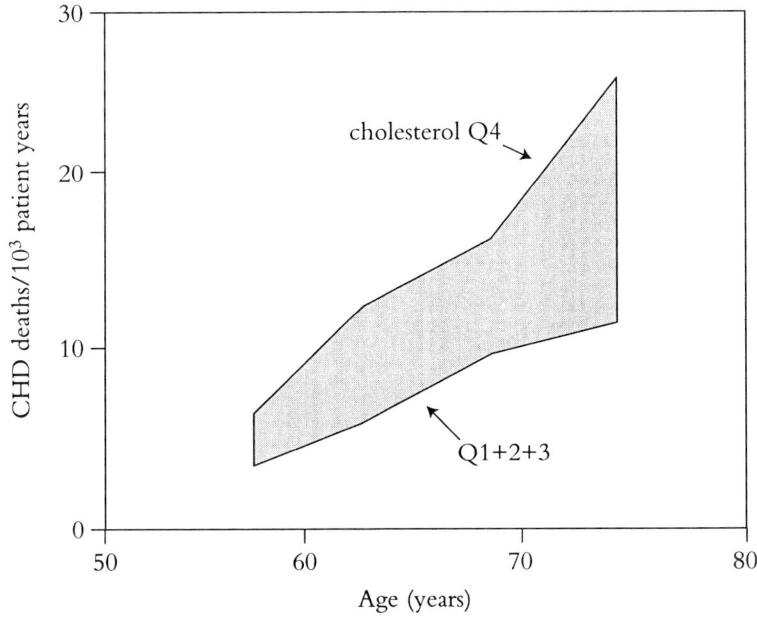

Figure 3 The excess of CHD deaths among individuals in the highest quartile of serum cholesterol over those in the other three quartiles increases with advancing age

The wide range of coronary risk factors assessed included TC and HDL cholesterol, and serum iron and albumen were measured as indices of debility. During data collection in the first year of study, 44 individuals died from CHD, and up to 1992, 208 further deaths occurred.

Plotting unadjusted relative risk of CVD events against TC in these elderly patients suggests that a higher cholesterol level was associated with a lower relative risk. However, successively adjusting for risk factors including debility, and excluding the individuals who died very early and were not followed for long, the negative association between cholesterol and risk becomes a strong positive one ($p = 0.005$). This would suggest that TC may well be a risk factor for CHD and death in the elderly, and that co-morbidity may confuse the relationships. However, much further work will be needed to clarify these points.

Does lipid lowering benefit the elderly in practice?

Evidence that treating hypercholesterolemia in the elderly is of clinical value comes from the major event-related coronary prevention trials already mentioned, 4S and CARE.

At the end of 4S, subjects of 61–75 years benefited from the treatment to the extent of a 29% reduction in relative risk. In absolute terms, seven individuals were saved for every 100 treated, and 14.7 subjects had to be treated over the five years of the study in order to avoid one event. The CARE study results were very similar. In people of 61–80 years, relative risk reduction from treatment was 27%, and the number to be treated over five years to avoid one event was 14.5 (Table 1).

Thus, lipid-lowering treatment with an HMG CoA reductase inhibitor represented reasonably good value for money in these studies. But it is important to note that not only was CHD avoided; for every 1000 elderly subjects in the CARE study who were treated for 5 years, 27 coronary deaths, 46 MI, 52 CABG or percutaneous transluminal coronary angioplasty (PTCA) operations, 25 strokes and 57 other CVD-related events were prevented. This is important because of the major use of acute medical services that such events represent (Table 2).

THE FUTURE

Since elevated serum cholesterol contributes to more CVD morbidity and mortality in the elderly than the young, lipid-lowering treatment resulting

Table 1 Risk reductions for all CVD events (and for deaths in the 4S study), and numbers of subjects treated with HMG CoA reductase inhibitors for five years to avoid one event, in the 4S and CARE studies[11,12]

		Risk reduction (%)		
Study	*Age*	*Relative*	*Absolute*	*Number treated to avoid one event**
4S	61–75	29	6.8	14.7
		27[†]	3.5[†]	28.6[†]
CARE	61–80	27	6.9	14.5

*, over 5 years; [†], deaths

Table 2 CVD-related events avoided among every 1000 individuals over 60 years (maximum 80 years) treated with HMG CoA reductase inhibitors for five years in the Cholesterol And Recent Events (CARE) study[12]

Events	Number avoided
CHD death	27
Nonfatal MI	46
CABG/PTCA	52
Stroke/TIA	25
Other CVD events	57
All CVD events	207

CHD, coronary heart disease; MI, myocardial infarction; CABG, coronary artery bypass grafting; PTCA, percutaneous transluminal coronary angioplasty; TIA, transient ischemic attack

in a small percentage reduction in mortality among that elderly group will translate into a large saving in life. However, this strategy, if it is to be pursued, should target not only CHD but also stroke, which is one of the major problems facing the elderly in the community, and one that is increasing year by year. In addition to massive strokes, minor strokes can lead to debility and dementia. It may actually be possible in future to prevent strokes and multi-infarct dementia by anticholesterolemic treatment. Of particular relevance here is the reduction in stroke incidence demonstrated in the 4S and CARE studies. Remarkably, this benefit not only approaches that achievable by antihypertensive therapy, but is also additive to it[18]. In view of this, perhaps now is the time to re-evaluate preventive strategies for cerebrovascular disease.

Finally, are we trying to avoid mortality, to help these elderly people live longer, or to help them live with a better quality of life? The answers to this question are complicated by another: are the cost implications of treatment going to be weighted on the beneficial side – is treatment really worthwhile? Only intervention studies with real-time cost/benefit analyses can lead us to a conclusion.

REFERENCES

1. Schultz, K.-L. and Beil, S. (1996). Efficacy and tolerability of fluvastatin and simvastatin in hypercholesterolaemic patients. *Clin. Drug Invest.*, **12**, 119–26

2. Shepherd, J., Cobbe, S. M., Ford, I., *et al.* (1995). Prevention of coronary heart disease with pravastatin in men with hypercholesterolemia. *N. Engl. J. Med.*, **333**, 1301–7

3. Furberg, C. D., Adams, H. P., Applegate, W. B., *et al.* (1994). Effect of lovastatin on early carotid atherosclerosis and cardiovascular events (ACAPS). *Circulation*, **90**, 1679–87

4. Waters, D., Higginson, L., Wadstone, P., *et al.* (1994). Effects of monotherapy with an HMG CoA reductase inhibitor on the progression of coronary atherosclerosis as assessed by serial quantitative arteriography (CCAIT). *Circulation*, **89**, 959–68

5. Blankenhorn, D. H., Azen, S. P., Kramsch, D. M., *et al.* (1993). Coronary angiographic changes with lovastatin therapy (MARS). *Ann. Intern. Med.*, **119**, 969–76

6. Salonen, R., Nyyssonen, K., Parkkala, E., *et al.* (1995). Kuopio atherosclerosis prevention study (KAPS). *Circulation*, **92**, 1758–64

7. Pitt, B., Ellis, S. G., Mancini, G. B. J., *et al.* (1993). Design and recruitment in the United States of a multicenter quantitative angiographic trial of pravastatin to limit atherosclerosis in the coronary arteries (PLAC I). *Am. J. Cardiol.*, **72**, 31–5

8. Crouse, J. R., Byington, R. P., Bond, M. G., *et al.* (1995). Pravastatin, lipids and atherosclerosis in the carotid arteries (PLAC II). *Am. J. Cardiol.*, **75**, 455–9

9. Jukema, J. W., Bruschke, A. V.G., van Boven, A. J., *et al.* (1995). Effects of lipid lowering by pravastatin on progression and regression of coronary artery disease in symptomatic men with normal to moderately elevated serum cholesterol levels (REGRESS). *Circulation*, **91**, 2528–40

10. MAAS Investigators. (1994). Effects of simvastatin on coronary atheroma: the multicenter antiatheroma study (MAAS). *Lancet*, **344**, 633–8

11. Scandinavian Simvastatin Survival Study Group. (1994). Ramdomised trial of cholesterol lowering in 4444 patients with coronary heart disease. *Lancet*, **344**, 1383–9

12. Sacks, F. M., Pfeffer, M. A., Moye, L. A., *et al.* (1996). The effect of pravastatin on coronary events after myocardial infarction in patients with average cholesterol levels. *N. Engl. J. Med.*, **335**, 1001–9

13. Shepherd, J. (1997). Pleiotropism among the statins. *Br. J. Cardiol.*, **4** (Suppl. 1), 528–31

14. Rifkind, B. M. and Segal, P. (1983). Lipid Research Clinics Program reference values of hyperlipidemia. *J. Am.Med.Assoc.*, **250**, 1869–72

15. Khan, K.-T. and Rose, G. (1989). Cholesterol screening programs: how much potential benefit? *Br. Med. J.*, **299**, 606–7

16. Shipley, M. J., Pocock, S. J. and Marmot, M. G. (1991). Does plasma cholesterol concentration predict mortality from coronary heart disease in elderly people? 18-year follow-up in the Whitehall study. *B. Med. J.*, **303**, 89–92

17. Corti, M.-C., Guralnik, J. M., Salive, M. E., *et al.* (1997). Clarifying the direct relation between total cholesterol levels and death from coronary heart disease in older persons. *Ann. Int. Med.*, **126**, 753–60

18. The West of Scotland Coronary Prevention Study Group. (1996). Clinical implications of the West of Scotland Coronary Prevention Study (WOSCOPS): identification of high risk groups and comparison with other cardiovascular intervention trials. *Lancet*, **348**, 1339–42

9

Cost-effectiveness approach to cardiovascular interventions in the elderly

L. H. Beck

INTRODUCTION

In a time of scarce resources for healthcare, it is important for individuals, health systems and society to ensure that interventions provide real benefit in terms of desired health outcomes. Increasing availability of costly technologies demands that we measure the value of such technologies before adopting them as standard practice. This is particularly true when considering clinical strategies for health problems in the elderly. The enormous growth of the elderly population, coupled with their limited remaining years of life and the increased potential for iatrogenic harm, makes such analysis crucial if we are to gain the optimal benefit from a limited healthcare budget.

Economic analysis of new strategies can be utilized to measure the value of such approaches and to compare them with those already in operation. Value in healthcare is defined as quality/cost, with quality usually measured as a desired health outcome. The latter is not necessarily the same when assessing value for patients of differing ages. Whereas 5- or 10-year survival may be an appropriate outcome measure for young and middle-aged individuals, for the elderly the more appropriate measure may be functional status, or quality-adjusted life years.

Despite recent decreases in the incidence of coronary heart disease in the American population, perhaps due in part to changes in life-style, heart disease remains an enormous problem in terms of health status and cost. It is estimated that the annual direct cost of care in the United States for coronary artery disease alone is about $17 billion. It is therefore crucial to define the most cost-effective and appropriate strategies for management of these patients.

When choosing whether to utilize a particular management strategy for elderly individuals (or for a population of such individuals), one should ask a series of questions:

(1) Is there a demonstrated health benefit?

(2) Does this benefit persist with increasing age?

(3) What is the cost of the strategy, and what outcomes are achieved for that cost? (cost-effectiveness)

(4) How does this cost-effectiveness compare with alternative strategies?

(5) What are the downstream effects on cost and quality of life?

Economic analysis of healthcare has become increasingly prevalent and important, particularly in the evaluation of the value of new drugs, procedures or other interventions[1]. The two principal techniques used are cost-effectiveness analysis (CEA) and cost–benefit analysis (CBA). Cost-effectiveness analysis is intrinsically more straightforward and more easily understood; it is the approach which will be used in this paper.

Cost-effectiveness is a measure of economic efficiency. It addresses the question: compared to the next best alternative, are the outcomes expected of a strategy worth the necessary investment of resources?

Cost-effectiveness is usually reported as a ratio:

$$\text{C/E ratio} = \frac{\text{Cost (a)} - \text{Cost (b)}}{\text{Effect (a)} - \text{Effect (b)}}$$

When considering interventions that prolong survival, many in the United States consider an intervention with a C/E ratio of less than $50 000/life-year to be 'cost-effective'.

Cost–benefit analysis, on the other hand, asks the question: does the intervention produce a net cost or a net saving? In CBA economic impact is the only scale used, so that a monetary value must be placed on the outcome variable (e.g. what is the economic value of a year of life gained?). Cost–benefit analysis is particularly problematic in assessing interventions in the elderly, because the strict economic value (in terms of remaining earning potential) would result in assigning little or no value to a year of life. This discussion will be limited, therefore, to the issue of cost-effectiveness, which is less subjective and easier to apply to the elderly population.

CARDIOVASCULAR INTERVENTIONS

The following two interventions will be discussed as examples of competing strategies: revascularization of occluded coronary arteries in elderly patients with established coronary artery disease, and primary or secondary prevention of coronary disease using lipid-lowering agents. Emphasis will be on the difficulty in developing global guidelines due to: 1) inadequate data on effectiveness of these interventions in elderly patients, and 2) difficulties related to using standard outcome measures and costs.

Since the early studies of Wennberg and others[2,3] it has been repeatedly demonstrated that there is dramatic regional variation in the utilization or delivery of specific health services, whether one compares countries with one another, or examines different regions within a single country. There are a number of possible reasons for such variation:

(1) Differences in severity of disease between populations;

(2) Availability of resources or of the technology in question;

(3) Cost (or perceived cost) of the service;

(4) Uncertainty of the medical benefit of the service; and

(5) Regional differences in patient preferences (e.g. are New Englanders more risk-averse than Californians?).

REVASCULARIZATION TECHNIQUES

In the United States each year more than 1 million coronary angiograms are performed. These result in about 400 000 angioplasties and a similar number of coronary artery bypass graft (CABG) operations. The GUSTO-1 trial (Global Utilization of Streptokinase and Tissue Plasminogen Activator for Occluded Coronary Arteries) was a multinational randomized controlled trial of 40 861 patients with myocardial infarction treated within six hours of onset of chest pain[4]. An analysis of American utilization patterns revealed a marked regional variation in the use of procedures[5]. For example, 81 per cent of eligible individuals received angiography in the south central region, as compared with 52 per cent in New England. In general, the use of procedures was directly related to the availability of cardiac care facilities in the regions. Despite the large regional differences, the frequency of use of angioplasty did not affect mortality or functional status outcomes, which were similar across all regions.

There were even more dramatic differences in utilization between the US and non-US participants[6]. Thirty-one per cent and 13 per cent of participants received angioplasty and CABG, respectively, in the US, compared to 10 per cent and 3 per cent in the non-US centers. Despite these differences, 30-day mortality was similar at about 7 per cent.

Similarly in the SAVE (Survival and Ventricular Enlargement) study, Rouleau reported on the utilization of these technologies between the 93 US and 19 Canadian centers which participated[7]. In the US 78 per cent of subjects had angiography, compared with 48 per cent in Canada. Large differences occurred also in utilization of percutaneous transluminal coronary angioplasty (PTCA) (27 per cent US versus 11 per cent Canadian) and CABG (22 per cent US versus 13 per cent Canadian). Once again, there was no difference in the measured outcome: survival or recurrent myocardial infarction. There was significantly less activity-limiting angina pectoris in the US patients in the study.

Owing to the large costs involved in either intervention, several studies have addressed the comparative outcomes and costs between PTCA and CABG after acute myocardial infarction. The RITA (Randomized Intervention Treatment of Angina) was a United Kingdom study that randomly assigned 1011 eligible patients to either PTCA or CABG[8]. At two years of follow-up, there was no difference in mortality or non-fatal myocardial infarction between the two interventions. There was a difference in subsequent angina (31 per cent in PTCA versus 21 per cent in CABG).

EAST (Emory Angioplasty versus Surgery Trial) was a similar randomized trial with assignment to PTCA or CABG carried out at a single large institution involving 392 patients with a mean age of 62 years[9]. Outcome measures included death, Q wave myocardial infarction and large reversible thallium scan defect. Functional status measures included per cent return to work and self-rated health status. There was no difference between the two procedures in any of these outcomes. There was a difference in subsequent procedures and recurrent angina: at 3 years, 23 per cent of the PTCA group had a repeat PTCA or CABG, versus only 14 per cent in the original CABG group.

Although the initial costs of the two procedures differ markedly, the increase in subsequent procedures in PTCA patients tended to bring these costs together. In EAST, the average cost at 3 years was \$23 734 for PTCA patients and \$25 320 for CABG[9]. Similarly in RITA, after 2 years the PTCA group costs had risen to equal about 80 per cent of those expended on the CABG group[8].

In summary, when measured over time, the two procedures are nearly equivalent in direct medical costs. The slightly lower cost for PTCA is offset by an increase in recurrent angina and need for repeated procedures.

None of the above studies calculated costs for those patients who received medical therapy alone. As noted, the regional variation studies cited previously suggest that the medical outcomes were in general similar in medically treated patients, and it is probable that their costs were less. Of the cited studies, only GUSTO specifically addressed the issue of intervention in the elderly[10]. When stratified by age, the outcomes for 30-day mortality, stroke and the combined outcome (death or non-fatal disabling cerebrovascular accident (CVA)) were all worse with increasing age (Table 1).

One of the principal purposes of GUSTO was to compare the use of tissue plasminogen activator (TPA) with streptokinase. With respect to mortality and disabling stroke, TPA was slightly better than streptokinase (odds ratio for the combined outcome was 0.8) in all age groups except those over 85. The investigators calculated the cost–effectiveness ratios for the two approaches and reported that for individuals over 75 years with anterior infarction, TPA cost \$13 410 per additional year of life saved (compared with \$49 877 for those aged 41–60 years), indicating an improved value of TPA with increasing age[11].

PRIMARY AND SECONDARY PREVENTION

As mentioned above, the cost of cardiac care is staggering, and a large proportion of that cost (in the United States at least) is in revascularization, the opening or bypassing of arteries occluded by cholesterol-rich

Table 1 Outcome for 30-day mortality, stroke, death or non-fatal disabling cerebrovascular accident with increasing age

Age (years)	*< 65*	*65–74*	*75–85*	*> 85*
30-day mortality (%)	3.0	9.5	19.5	30.3
Stroke (%)	0.8	2.1	3.4	2.9
Death or non-fatal disabling CVA (%)	3.3	10.2	20.5	33.1

CVA, cerebrovascular accident

atherosclerotic plaques. A more attractive approach to coronary artery disease, for individuals and for society, would be prevention, primary or secondary, thereby avoiding the high cost of 'damage repair'.

Life style changes can certainly be effective in decreasing the incidence of coronary disease, but compliance is often difficult. Numerous studies have shown the value of primary and secondary prevention using lipid-lowering drugs. From the financial standpoint, however, widespread use of these drugs presents a fiscal conundrum. Costs are loaded up front for benefits that are realized several years downstream. Governments, health systems and even individuals are often reluctant to spend money this year when the health benefit and fiscal return (in terms of cost avoidance) will not be achieved right away.

As with revascularization, it is appropriate to apply the series of economic and health benefit questions listed previously to determine if widespread diagnostic testing and treatment of hypercholesterolemia in the elderly is appropriate (and cost-effective). Numerous large well-designed studies published in the last 5 years have demonstrated the dramatic effects of lipid-lowering agents, in particular the hydroxymethylglutaryl coenzyme A (HMG CoA) reductase inhibitors ('statins') in the primary and secondary prevention of myocardial infarction and cardiovascular death. The West of Scotland study enrolled 6595 men with hypercholesterolemia (cholesterol > 252 mg/dl; mean level 272 mg/dl) to receive 40 mg pravastatin or placebo each evening[12]. The primary outcomes were non-fatal myocardial infarction and death from coronary artery disease. After an average follow-up of 5 years, the pravastatin group showed dramatic results: 31 per cent fewer non-fatal myocardial infarctions and a 28 per cent reduction in coronary death. Furthermore, there was a 22 per cent reduction in death from any cause.

Similarly, randomized trials using lipid-lowering agents in patients following first myocardial infarction have demonstrated reductions in rates of recurrent myocardial infarction and in death from cardiovascular disease. The Scandinavian Simvastatin Survival Study (4S) randomized over 4000 patients with elevated cholesterol following myocardial infarction, and demonstrated a 37 per cent reduction in coronary events in the simvastatin-treated group after 4.9 years[13]. Furthermore, the Cholesterol and Recurrent Events (CARE) trial, published recently, evaluated the effect of pravastatin on men and postmenopausal women with recent myocardial infarction who did not have marked hyperlipidemia (total cholesterol at entry less than

240 mg/dl; mean level 209 mg/dl)[14]. At 5 years of follow-up, the treatment group had experienced a 24 per cent reduction in fatal coronary events or non-fatal myocardial infarction (absolute risk reduction was from 13.2 to 10.2 per cent in the pravastatin group).

Unfortunately, these studies have rarely addressed the value of preventive interventions specifically in the elderly. The West of Scotland Study did not enroll men over the age of 64 years. The CARE trial, on the other hand, did not set age criteria. Mean age was 59 years, and subsequent analysis showed no difference in effectiveness for those over or under 60 years of age (although there were few patients over the age of 75).

In part because of lack of clear evidence of benefit of lipid-lowering therapy in the elderly, national guidelines, such as those of the Untied States Preventive Services Task Force and the Canadian Task Force, recommend routine cholesterol screening only until 65 years of age and are ambivalent about the value of screening and treatment over the age of 65. Garber *et al.* estimated that if the NCEP (National Cholesterol Education Program) recommendations were uniformly applied to 'asymptomatic' Americans over the age of 65, the total cost for screening or treatment would exceed $16 billion in 1990 dollars[15]. Since there were inadequate data available concerning outcomes of such a strategy in the elderly, they did not perform a cost-effectiveness analysis. However, it is interesting to note that this estimated cost is very similar to the current direct medical costs of coronary artery disease cited above.

A number of authors have calculated cost-effectiveness ratios for primary and secondary prevention using a variety of lipid-lowering agents and outcome data from earlier trials. One of the most extensive analyses was published by Goldman *et al.* who used a computer simulation, the Coronary Heart Disease Policy Model, to project cost-effectiveness of lovastatin in men and women aged 35–84 years who are at risk of developing coronary disease or who have experienced a first coronary event[16]. The model allowed stratification by age range as well as by various risk factors (level of serum cholesterol, diastolic blood pressure, and smoking status).

Goldman *et al.* used a value of $40 000 as a threshold, suggesting that cost per year of life gained below that value might be an acceptable societal cost. (For comparison, the estimated cost of renal dialysis in 1989 was $35 000 to $40 000 per year, an expense which the United States has been willing to pay.) The estimated cost per year of life saved when lovastatin was used as secondary prevention ranged from $10 000 to $38 000 for men over 65 years, depending on the dose of lovastatin employed (20 mg or 40 mg). When a program of primary prevention was superimposed, however, the cost per year saved was greater than $40 000 per year in virtually all risk groups. For men over 65 years, cost per year of life saved was less than $40 000 if limited to those with severe concomitant hypertension. For normotensive elderly men, the values were prohibitive, ranging from $85 000 to $210 000 per year of life saved. The reasons for these very high costs per year of life gained are the high prevalence of disease and high incidence of coronary events in the elderly, coupled with the shortened expected survival.

An economic analysis of the 4S data was recently published, in which the authors estimated the cost per year of life gained for different subsets of patients encountered in that trial[17]. The three variables used to stratify the population were gender, age and serum cholesterol levels. In this secondary prevention trial, cost-effectiveness ratios were acceptable for all age groups, and ranged from a low of $3800 (in men aged 70 with serum cholesterol > 300 mg/dl) to a peak of $27 400 (in women aged 35 with serum cholesterol of 213 mg/dl). For elderly men and women (aged 70) the cost per year of life gained ranged from $3800 to $13 300. If United States drug acquisition and treatment costs are substituted for the Swedish costs, these trial-derived estimates are quite similar to those predicted by the Goldman model for secondary prevention.

Cost-effectiveness and cost–benefit analyses involving elderly patients are decidedly more complex than the above studies would suggest for at least two reasons:

(1)   The reality of competing mortality risks; and

(2)   The issue of 'compression of morbidity'.

To the extent that any intervention results in decreased cardiovascular mortality or overall mortality, the elderly individual becomes exposed to the competing risk of other age-associated illness, such as cancer or degenerative disease. These conditions will require the expenditure of resources that would have been 'avoided' had the individual succumbed to the cardiovascular disease. These types of 'induced' costs, which contribute to the overall societal healthcare expenditures, are difficult to model and have rarely been included in economic analyses of healthcare strategies for the elderly.

The second complicating factor is even more difficult to model, but it too is related to the issue of competing risks. Many geriatricians argue that the goal of any intervention in elderly patients should be to delay and compress the period of severe morbidity, so that the length of time in a state of disability is minimized prior to death. This goal aims not only at maintaining the highest possible functional status, but also at controlling healthcare costs at the end of life. This is of particular concern with those interventions that actually decrease overall mortality and extend life. Few studies that demonstrate an effect on mortality have evaluated whether morbidity is simultaneously compressed or expanded, or whether the downstream costs have been affected.

With respect to the effect of prolongation of survival on health-related costs in the elderly, however, two recent US studies have reported encouraging results. As would be expected, lifetime Medicare expenditures increase with increasing age at death ($13 044 for those who die at age 65 [the first year of eligibility for Medicare]; $56 094 if death occurs at age 80)[18]. However, the payment associated with an additional year of life progressively decreases with increasing age, so that total costs tend to flatten out beyond 80 years of age.

In another analysis of Medicare recipients in Massachusetts, the average cost of hospitalization decreased in very old patients, after peaking in the 70 to 79 years age range[19]. For patients who died, hospital costs decreased, from about $17 000 per final hospital stay for 60–69-year-olds, to about $6500 per final hospital stay for centenarians. When these observations are coupled with current data on improved life expectancy for the elderly US population, the effect of increased longevity on overall Medicare spending per individual becomes trivial. Whether these same projections can apply to the years of life gained for primary and/or secondary prevention strategies in the elderly is unknown.

A final issue to be considered is a purely economic one. Under conditions of scarce resources, in order to incorporate additional healthcare services, other areas of resource utilization should be curtailed. As pointed out by Gafni[20], to implement a new intervention that results in improved outcomes, but at a higher cost, some other intervention(s) need(s) to be eliminated in order to provide the necessary resources for the new one. Although it is easy to suggest that such resources might be found in the global healthcare budget (e.g. by eliminating 'waste'), a more appropriate (and stringent) requirement would be to allow adoption of a new strategy only if the necessary resources could be generated from current strategies aimed at the same health problem (e.g. coronary artery disease).

CONCLUSION

With respect to choosing the widespread adoption for elderly patients of either or both of the two types of interventions used as models in this paper, let us return to the series of questions posed at the beginning.

(1) Is there a demonstrated health benefit?

    (a) For revascularization, the benefit (when compared to medical therapy) is real, as measured in terms of decreased myocardial infarction and relief of angina.

    (b) For primary and secondary treatment of hypercholesterolemia, there is clear evidence that cardiovascular events are reduced and survival is improved.

(2) Does the benefit accrue to all age groups?

    (a) Revascularization has been used extensively in the elderly population, but it is unclear if there is a benefit, in terms of morbidity and mortality, compared to medical therapy. It is clear that morbidity and mortality associated with these procedures rise dramatically with increasing age, but it is uncertain whether these outcomes are different from similarly aged patients not receiving revascularization.

    (b) With respect to treatment of hypercholesterolemia for primary or secondary prevention, the available data on the elderly are generally limited. Such studies need to be carried out if we are to make evidence-based decisions on care.

(3) What is the cost-effectiveness of the strategy?

    (a) As reviewed, the cumulative costs are quite similar between angioplasty and coronary artery bypass graft. However, these have not been compared directly to similar patients receiving medical therapy alone, so the incremental cost-effectiveness of either intervention is unknown.

(b) For treatment of hypercholesterolemia, estimates of cost-effectiveness have been made but have been limited by the paucity of outcome data in those over 65 years. It does appear, however, that except in selected groups with additional risk factors, primary prevention would become 'prohibitively' expensive (in terms of cost per year of life gained) if applied universally to very old individuals.[a]

(4) How does the cost-effectiveness compare with alternative strategies?

(a) As noted above, this comparison has not been made for revascularization procedures.

(b) For treatment of hypercholesterolemia, the cost per year of life compares favorably with other 'accepted' strategies only in selected elderly individuals.[a]

(5) What are the downstream effects on costs and quality of life?

As discussed above, this is a virtually unexplored area, particularly in the aged population. Although survival benefits have been demonstrated, in particular for treatment of hypercholesterolemia, it is unclear whether such prolongation will result in a net benefit for elderly individuals in terms of quality of life, in view of the competing risks that they will then encounter. For those with added life-years, will morbidity be compressed or expanded?

Finally, with increasing recognition of the 'ceiling' which is being approached (or already reached) in healthcare resource expenditure, how will governments, health plans, or other decision-making bodies decide between cost-effective strategies? Although the economic approaches reviewed in this paper can help to identify and clarify the alternatives and trade-offs, making the choice between alternatives will become one of the major challenges of the next decade.

---

[a]The cost-effectiveness (and, therefore, affordability) of primary cholesterol screening and management in the elderly could increase markedly if newer pharmacological agents are shown to be much more effective, or if competition and/or improved production techniques were to decrease costs significantly.

REFERENCES

1. Eisenberg, J. M. (1989). Clinical economics: a guide to the economic analysis of clinical practices. *J. Am. Med. Assoc.*, **262**, 2879–86

2. Wennberg, J. and Gittelsohn, A. (1973). Small area variations in health care delivery. *Science*, **182**, 1102–8

3. Wennberg, J. E., Freeman, J. L., Shelton, R. M., *et al.* (1989). Hospital use and mortality among Medicare beneficiaries in Boston and New Haven. *N. Engl. J. Med.*, **321**, 1168–73

4. The GUSTO Investigators. (1993). An international randomized trial comparing four thrombolytic strategies for acute myocardial infarction. *N. Engl. J. Med.*, **329**, 673–82

5. Pilote, L., Califf, R. M., Sapp, S., *et al.* (1995). Regional variation across the United States in the management of acute myocardial infarction. *N. Engl. J. Med.*, **333**, 565–72

6. Van de Werf, F., Topol, E. J., Lee, K. L., *et al.* (1995). Variations in patient management and outcomes for acute myocardial infarction in the United States and other countries. *J. Am. Med. Assoc.*, **273**, 1586–91

7. Rouleau, J. L., Moye, L. A., Pfeffer, M. A., *et al.* (1993). A comparison of management patterns after acute myocardial infarction in Canada and the United States. *N. Engl. J. Med.*, **328**, 779–84

8. Sculpher, M. J., Seed, P. and Henderson, R. A. (1994). Health service costs of coronary angioplasty and coronary artery bypass surgery: the Randomized Intervention Treatment of Angina (RITA) Trial. *Lancet*, **344**, 927–30

9. Weintraub, W. S., Mauldin, P. D., Becker, E., *et al.* (1995). Comparison of the costs and quality of life after coronary angioplasty or coronary surgery for multivessel coronary artery disease: results from the Emory Angioplasty Surgery Trial (EAST). *Circulation*, **92**, 2831–40

10. White, H. D., Barbesh, G. I., Califf, R. M., *et al.* (1996). Age and outcome with contemporary thrombolytic therapy. Results from the GUSTO-1 trial. *Circulation*, **94**, 1826–33

11. Mark, D. B., Hlatky, M. A. and Califf, R. M. (1995). Cost effectiveness of thrombolytic therapy with tissue plasminogen activator as compared with streptokinase for acute myocaridal infarction. *N. Engl. J. Med*, **332**, 1418–24

12. Shepherd, J., Cobbe, S. M. and Ford, I. (1995). Prevention of coronary heart disease with pravastatin in men with hypercholesterolemia. *N. Engl. J. Med.*, **333**, 1301–7

13. Scandinavian Simvastatin Survival Study Group. (1994). Randomized trial of cholesterol lowering in 4444 patients with coronary heart disease: the Scandinavian Simvastatin Survival Study (4S). *Lancet*, **344**, 1383–9

14. Sacks, F. M., Pfeffer, M. A., Moye, L. A., *et al.* (1996). The effect of pravastatin on coronary events after myocardial infarction in patients with average cholesterol levels. *N. Engl. J. Med.*, **335**, 1001–9

15. Garber, A. M., Littenberg, B., Sox, H. C., *et al.* (1991) Costs and health consequences of cholesterol screening for asymptomatic older Americans. *Arch. Intern. Med.*, **151**, 1089–95

16. Goldman, L., Weinstein, M. C., Goldman, P. A., *et al.* (1991). Cost-effectiveness of HMG-CoA reductase inhibition for primary and secondary prevention of coronary heart disease. *J. Am. Med. Assoc*, **265**, 1145–51

17. Johannesson, M., Jonsson, B., Kjekshus, J., *et al.* (1997). Cost effectiveness of simvastatin treatment to lower cholesterol levels in patients with coronary heart disease. *N. Engl. J. Med.*, **336**, 332–6

18. Lubitz, J., Beebe, J. and Baker, C. (1995). Longevity and Medicare expenditures. *N. Engl. J. Med.*, **332**, 999–1003

19. Perls, T. T. and Wood, E. R. (1996). Acute care costs of the oldest old. *Arch Intern. Med.*, **156**, 754–60

20. Gafni, A. (1996). Economic evaluation of health care interventions: an economist's perspective. *ACP Journal Club*, **124**, A 12–14

Summary

E. G. Lakatta

Coronary artery disease (CAD) prevalence and mortality rates vary widely among countries, and in all countries, CAD rates are 3- to 4-fold higher in men than in women. Advanced age is the most potent risk factor for CAD, i.e. the same level of most standard risk factors, e.g. plasma lipid or blood pressure conferring the highest quintile risk for CAD in younger persons is equivalent to the lowest quintile risk in older persons. Whether this increased risk of CAD in older persons is the result of prolonged exposure to these risk factors, or is a reflection of a change in the biology of the organism intrinsic to the aging process, is not yet known with certainty. In support of the latter, experimental data indicate that the response to a defined atherogenic stimulus becomes exaggerated with increasing age.

In most countries substantial declines in CAD mortality rates in both sexes have occurred during the past few decades, although notable exceptions are central and eastern European countries and some Asian countries, such as Singapore. In western countries, most postponed deaths have occurred in older persons (75 and over), and women have benefited more than men in these favorable trends, as reflected in the continuing gap in life expectancy between men and women. However, these favorable trends in CAD mortality rates are offset by global demographic trends for an increase in life expectancy, and the resultant increase in the number of older individuals within a society will have the effect of increasing the absolute number of individuals with CAD. This worldwide increase in life expectancy will continue to have the greatest impact in the Asian continent, and by the year 2025, six of the top ten nations worldwide with the greatest number of older persons (> 60 years old) will be Asian countries. In many Asian countries there is a relative lack of information on mortality rates for CAD in older persons, owing to a paucity of epidemiological studies considering CAD as the main endpoint.

The link of well known risk factors, i.e. age, diet, plasma cholesterol, physical activity and smoking, to the likelihood for clinical CAD occurrence that has been well established in western countries, is now dramatically exemplified in some Asian countries in which marked increases in CAD have begun to occur. For example, Singapore, which has the second fastest growing aging society in the world, a fact that aggravates the CAD problem, has overtaken Australia in having the highest mortality rate from ischemic heart disease in the eastern Pacific. In Singapore, the mortality rate from ischemic heart disease is greatest among the Indian subset of the population, their rate being about twice that of other ethnic contingents. Epidemiological surveys seem to unequivocally indicate that the marked increase in the prevalence of CAD is linked to the worsening of the risk factor profiles in Singapore. For example, between 1960 and 1985, the percentage of calories from meat and egg fat in the diet of the Singaporeans increased enormously and their average serum cholesterol ranks fifth highest in the world. Physical activity has decreased in women, while the incidence of obesity has increased and smoking has sharply increased. In contrast to Singapore, the incidence of CAD in China is the lowest among multi-population comparisons, but the incidence of stroke is higher. The fact that Chinese in Hong Kong have a higher incidence of CAD than stroke may be explained in part by the influence of the aforementioned effects of lifestyle on the risk for CAD.

While the majority of 'standard' risk factors for developing clinical CAD at younger ages are also relevant in older persons, the relative magnitude and risk potency of some factors change with aging, and age/gender issues emerge. Systolic blood pressure continues to increase in both men and women until about 80 years of age. Hypertension, because of its high prevalence and sustained impact with advancing age, particularly elevated systolic blood pressure, emerges as the dominant risk factor for CAD in older individuals of both genders. In fact, hypertension increases the absolute risk for clinical CAD to a greater extent in older than in younger persons. Total serum cholesterol peaks in men at about 60 years of age, but continues to increase in women until they are about 75 years old. High density lipoprotein (HDL) cholesterol in women is higher than in men across the life span, particularly in postmenopausal years, and only a modest decline in HDL cholesterol is associated with menopause. Still, women in the highest quintile of cholesterol have lower CAD rates than men in the lowest quintile, both pre- and postmenopausally. While CAD in women is increasingly depicted as being linked to menopause, there is no immediate increase in incidence at menopause; rather a graded increase in CAD occurs over the ensuing three to four decades. In some western countries, while hormone replacement therapy for the prevention of heart disease in menopausal women has become widespread, its effectiveness in preventing vascular disease is not yet unequivocally established.

Serum cholesterol as the sole measure of risk for CHD attributable to serum lipids should now be considered obsolete, based on current understanding of the impact of various lipoprotein subfractions and the availability of standardized laboratory methods to measure them in clinical practice. While the serum lipid fractions lose some statistical power as a predictor for CAD, particularly in older men, a consensus (though not unanimous) opinion is that elevated plasma lipids, particularly when confounding concomitant risk factors and co-morbidity are taken into account, still confer an increased risk for clinical events resulting from CAD in older persons (albeit with less impact than in younger persons). The current consensus also holds that elevated levels of serum triglycerides represent a risk marker for obesity, glucose intolerance and low HDL levels, all of which confer risk for CAD. However, a partially divergent view emerges from the Dubbo Study in Australia which shows that while elevated low density lipoprotein (LDL) cholesterol and triglyceride levels are significant predictors of CAD in older men and women aged 60–69 years, these lipids lack predictive power in both men and women aged 70 years and older. The presence of antecedent CAD remains an important predictor of CAD events in older persons, and serum lipids appear to be a more prominent risk factor in this context than hypertension.

Two types of prospective studies have been implemented to determine whether interventions that lower plasma cholesterol can decrease the CAD risk. One type employs angiography and ultrasound to detect evident changes in atherosclerotic lesions within arteries following drug treatment or placebo; the other type, in contrast, measures the efficacy of an intervention to reduce clinical CAD events, i.e. morbidity and mortality. These two endpoints are related but not synonymous. Several small scale, but important, invasive angiographical studies ('coronary regression trials') during the last decade have documented that a reduction in plasma lipids by HMG CoA reductase inhibitors, drugs which have a profound influence on plasma lipid and lipoprotein concentrations, mainly through a reduction of plasma LDL cholesterol of up to 35 per cent, and also via an increase in serum HDL cholesterol by up to 10 per cent can decrease the rate of progression, and, to a lesser extent, effect minor regression of the coronary atherosclerotic process. While meta-analyses of these several smaller studies reveal an overall favorable effect on clinical endpoints including total mortality, these unfortunately do not provide specific data with respect to older persons.

Considerable research is under way in several centers in North America and Europe to develop non-invasive techniques to detect and monitor the preclinical atherosclerotic vascular lesion. A recent trial (MARS) employing a non-invasive measurement of the carotid artery intimal medial thickness (IMT) as a study endpoint, observed that the expected age-associated increase in IMT is blunted by statin drugs and lifestyle changes. Other non-invasive techniques, notably magnetic resonance imaging and electron beam CT scanning (EBCT), have shown impressive sensitivity and specificity for identifying significant stenoses in the major coronary arteries, but accurate detection of early, pre-stenotic lesions still proves difficult using these techniques. The usefulness of EBCT is also being tested in screening patients for the presence and severity of coronary arterial calcification, a putative marker of coronary atherosclerosis.

Within the last two years, three major CAD event endpoint trials have been completed: the West of Scotland Coronary Prevention Study (WOSCOPS), a primary prevention trial in men only, the Scandinavian Simvastatin Survival Study (4S) and the Cholesterol And Recent Events (CARE) study. The latter two studies are secondary prevention trials, i.e. both men and women who participated had had a prior myocardial infarction. All three trials demonstrated a substantial (24–34 per cent) reduction in cardiovascular deaths and non-fatal myocardial infarctions over the course of about 5 years. Most interestingly, the fact that these benefits often become evident within a 6 month period suggests that the HMG CoA reductase inhibitors may reduce the frequency of CAD events through additional actions to that of lowering plasma lipids, i.e. via an anti-inflammatory effect, by 'normalizing' the arterial endothelium, stabilizing atherosclerotic plaques and by inhibiting lipoprotein oxidation or the formation of platelet-rich thrombi. Both the 4S and CARE studies demonstrated that the statin drugs do confer secondary prevention against CAD events in older individuals: persons aged 61–80 years showed a 29 per cent reduction in relative CAD risk. Unfortunately, the WOSCOP study did not enrol men over the age of 65 years and thus there are currently no data regarding primary prevention of CAD in older persons. A study in progress, the Anti-hypertensive and Lipid-lowering Treatment to Prevent Heart Attack Trial, which includes a sub-study of LDL-lowering in 20 000 older individuals, may provide needed data with respect to clinical events.

The foregoing summary of the generally limited data on the elderly from completed intervention trials, with respect to treatment of hypercholesterolemia for primary or secondary prevention, indicates that a strong case can be made for lipid intervention in older men and women aged 60 to 70 years, or perhaps to 80 years of age having established CAD. However, the case for lipid intervention in still older patients with established CAD remains problematic, but treatment and the case for cholesterol reduction in those aged 60 years and above, who are currently free of clinical CAD, remains unproven. Additional data are required for evidence-based decisions on whether to treat these individuals. There are two contrasting general strategies for prevention of CAD: the high risk (or individual) strategy and the population (or 'mass') strategy, the latter designed to reduce the average risk of CAD in the entire community. Most of the interventions which have been demonstrated to impact significantly on CAD have been applied at the population level, for example, smoking cessation, dietary changes and physical activity to reduce cholesterol, blood pressure levels and body weight. That global aging is a main driving force of the worldwide CAD epidemic which adversely changes the risk factor profiles of some populations, continues to render the population approach appealing.

It is critical that decisions as to whether to embark on lipid-lowering drug therapy in older individuals discriminate between the absolute risk of CAD, i.e. the number of older individuals likely to incur clinical CAD owing to the global increase in life expectancy and because age itself is a major risk factor for CAD, and the specific potency of a given risk factor, i.e. the relative risk it confers to a given older individual. Sole reliance on absolute risk as a criterion for intervention in the context of primary prevention will inevitably result in the eligibility for treatment of most men over the age of 70, whatever their serum cholesterol. This raises issues regarding cost- effectiveness, given that the relative potency of the risk of elevated plasma lipids in a given individual decreases with age. Thus, there is a considerable diversity of opinion regarding treatment strategies to lower risk factors for primary CAD in older persons: while the beneficial effect of treatment of hypercholesterolemia, as assessed by reduction in relative risk in older individuals, may be similar to or lower than that in younger ones, because of incidence and prevalence of CAD in older age groups, the same effect, when measured as a difference in absolute risk, reflecting reduction in numerical toll of disease outcomes, will actually remain higher in older persons. (A corollary of this phenomenon effect is that a smaller number of older vs. younger persons must be treated to yield the same prevention of disease event numbers.)

Estimates of the cost-effectiveness of lipid-lowering therapy for those over 65 years of age have been limited by the paucity of outcome data. Cost-effectiveness and cost–benefit analyses involving older patients are decidedly complex, because competing mortality risks and 'compression of morbidity' confound the issue. It is noteworthy that where cardiovascular or overall mortality is reduced in older individuals by lipid-lowering therapy, these individuals are still exposed to competing risk of other age-associated illness, probably requiring expenditures that would have been 'avoided' had the individual succumbed to CAD. These types of 'induced' health costs have rarely been included in economic analyses of lipid-lowering strategies for older persons, and are of particular concern regarding interventions that actually decrease overall mortality and extend life. Additionally, whether the effect of lowering lipids on CAD mortality simultaneously compresses or expands morbidity, or affects healthcare costs near the end of life, remains to be demonstrated. It does appear, however, that except in selected sub-groups at high risk, the primary prevention of CAD by lowering plasma lipids would become 'prohibitively' expensive (in terms of cost per year of life gained) if applied universally to very old individuals. The cost-effectiveness (and, therefore, affordability) of primary cholesterol screening and management in the elderly could increase markedly if novel, more effective pharmacological agents were designed, or if costs were to decrease significantly.

Based upon the albeit incomplete evidence outlined above, national and international organizations have issued age-associated guidelines on lipid-lowering therapy for older persons. These organizations concur that age, *per se*, is not a factor in the decision to treat elevated plasma lipids in individuals with known CAD, i.e. secondary prevention. However, attitudes differ regarding primary prevention, i.e. the treatment of elevated lipids in older persons who do not have, or who never have had, symptoms of CAD. For example, the European Atherosclerosis Society, the National Heart Foundation of New Zealand and the US National Cholesterol Education Program encourage primary prevention up to, or even after, the age of 75 years in asymptomatic individuals with hypercholesterolemia who are otherwise healthy and appear to have a reasonable life expectancy. In contrast, the British Hyperlipidaemia Association does not advocate lipid-lowering drug therapy after the age of 65 years. The American College of Physician's guidelines for screening (and by implication for treatment) discourage measuring serum cholesterol after 75 years of age, and question the benefits of doing so between 65 and 75 years. The joint guidelines of the European Society of Cardiology, European Atherosclerosis Society and European Society of Hypertension advocate treating hyperlipidemia up to the age of 70 years if the absolute risk of CAD exceeds 20–30 per cent per 10 years.

In conclusion, the world's population is aging, and the absolute number of older persons at risk for CAD, both those who have clinical CAD and those who are clinically asymptomatic but likely to have subclinical CAD (because age, *per se*, is the major risk factor for CAD), is increasing exponentially worldwide and thus results in an increase in the number of older individuals with CAD. This results in a substantial increase in the proportion of deaths from CAD between the ages of 65 and 75 years of age and the majority after the age of 75 years. Thus, any decision to undertake prevention of CAD in older individuals, if successful, would have major implications for the demography of death and also for health economics. While relative risk of an abnormal plasma lipid profile in a given older individual is less than in a younger one, elevated plasma LDL cholesterol still confers an enhanced risk for CAD in older individuals at least up to the age of 70 years. However, it is imperative that decisions to treat plasma lipids in older individuals are based on firm evidence of a beneficial and cost-effective outcome. While the current consensus of opinion is to treat elevated plasma lipids in older individuals who are already diagnosed as having CAD, in order to prevent a subsequent clinical event, i.e. secondary CAD prevention, there is no consensus regarding treatment of asymptomatic older individuals who have never had prior manifestations of CAD, i.e. primary CAD prevention. Given the present uncertain benefit from lipid-lowering therapy in these latter persons over the age of 65 years, divergent guidelines for the primary prevention of CAD in the elderly have been issued by several national and international organizations. There is an obvious need for a primary prevention trial of lipid-lowering therapy in subjects over the age of 65 years with CHD and total mortality as endpoints. However, confusion will continue to arise if clinical trials continue to utilize only clinical events to determine the impact of risk factors for a disease process that causes vascular lesions which can progress silently for decades in apparently healthy individuals, or erupt dramatically with minimal progression. Thus, there remains a great need to develop non-invasive techniques sufficiently sensitive to directly assess the vascular endpoint of risk factors, i.e. the presence of early atherosclerotic lesions and their progression. This direct evaluation of vascular endpoints in specific individuals would undoubtedly obviate the population or 'mass' approach to lifestyle and pharmacological interventions, and identify individuals at high risk at a sufficiently early stage to eradicate clinical CAD as we know it today.

Index

absolute risk 111–112
ACAPS study 119
adiposity 16
aging population
    Asian countries 55
        Singapore 60
    cardiovascular disease and 10–13,
        85–87
    risk factor changes 13–18, 121–122
alcohol consumption 46, 48, 50
    China, stroke incidence and 62, 63
    protective effect 77
ALLHAT (Anti-hypertensive and
    Lipid-lowering
        Treatment to Prevent Heart
        Attack Trial) 110
American College of Physicians
    (ACP) 111
angina pectoris 12, 26, 69, 91, 133
    age-related incidence 11
angiography 69, 92, 93–95, 97, 131
angioplasty 102, 131–132
antihypertensive drug therapy 22–23,
    46, 48, 50
    cardiovascular disease prevention
        34, 35, 49, 50, 81–82
    in women 73
aortic aneurysms 91, 92
arterial (aortic) compliance estimation
    92–94
arteriosclerosis 91, 92
Asian countries 55–70
    aging phenomenon 55
    causes of death 56–63
    impact of lifestyle changes 69–70
    see also individual countries

atherosclerosis 14, 29, 91
    plaque characterization 98
atorvastatin 101, 117

blood lipids *see* cholesterol;
    triglycerides
blood pressure
    age-related changes 13–15, 76
    risk associations for coronary heart
        disease 18, 19–23, 31–32, 43
    see also antihypertensive drug
        therapy; hypertension
body weight
    age-related changes 16
    reduction of 35
    risk associations for coronary heart
        disease 19, 29–30
    see also obesity
breast cancer 80, 83
breath-hold contrast-enhanced MRA
    92
British Hyperlipidaemia Association
    (BHA) 111

calcification, coronary artery 95–97
Canadian Task Force 135
cardiovascular diseases (CVD)
    in Asian countries 55–71
        as cause of death 56–63
        Japan 64, 65
        MONICA project 64
    in the elderly 10–11
    in women 74–75
    prevention strategies 74, 81–87

high-risk strategy 81–83
population strategy 81
primary and secondary
    prevention 133–138
sex differences 77–78
see also coronary heart disease;
    myocardial infarction; stroke
cardiovascular interventions 131
economic analysis 129–130
revascularization techniques
    131–133
see also lipid-lowering therapy
CARE (Cholesterol and Recurrent
    Events) Trial 49, 102, 110, 120,
    124, 125, 134–135
chest pain *see* angina pectoris
China 62–63
Chinese Stroke and Hypertension
    Surveys 62
cholesterol
    age-related changes 15–16
    Asian countries
        China 63
        Japan 67
        Singapore 61
    risk associations for coronary heart
        disease 19, 23–26, 43–44, 101
        Dubbo Study 44–48, 49, 50
        in the elderly 106–107, 121–123
        initial versus recurrent coronary
            disease 45–48
    sex differences 76–77
    synthesis inhibition 118–119
    see also high density lipoprotein
        cholesterol; lipid-lowering
        therapy; low density lipoprotein
        cholesterol
Churchill phenomenon 107
cigarette smoking
    age-related changes 17

cardiovascular disease prevention
    strategies 81
China, stroke incidence and 62, 63
risk associations for coronary heart
    disease 19, 26–27, 31, 43, 77
    passive smoking 77
Singapore 61
combined hypertension 15
compliance, arterial 92–94
computed tomography (CT) 92
    screening for coronary heart disease
        95–98
contrast-enhanced EBCT angiography
    97
contrast-enhanced spiral computed
    tomography 92
coronary arterial bypass graft (CABG)
    131–133
coronary artery calcification 95–97
coronary artery restenosis 102–103
coronary heart disease (CHD) 9–10
    antecedent CHD as predictor of
        future events 31–32
    in the elderly 10–13
        incidence 10–12
        manifestations of 12–13
        risk profiles 32–34
    menopause and 78–81
    mortality
        decline 34–35, 73, 76
        in women 74, 79
        international differences 75–76
    prediction of 43–48, 49–50
        Dubbo Study 44–48, 49, 50
        initial versus recurrent coronary
            disease 45–48
        left ventricular hypertrophy as
            predictor 29
        see also risk factors
    preventative measures 43, 49,
        101–103

absolute risk limitations as basis
  for therapeutic decisions
  111–112
interventional studies 49, 101
primary prevention strategies
  34–35, 109–111
see also antihypertensive drug
  therapy;
        lipid-lowering therapy
screening for using electron beam
  CT 95–98
sex differences 11–12
see also cardiovascular diseases
Coronary Heart Disease Policy Model
  135
coronary insufficiency 12
coronary regression trials 102
cost-benefit analysis (CBA) 130
cost-effectiveness analysis (CEA)
  130–139
  lipid-lowering therapy 134–138
  primary and secondary prevention
    133–138
  revascularization techniques
    131–133
Cox proportional hazards model 19

death *see* mortality; sudden death
Diabetes Control and Complications
  Trial 29
diabetes mellitus, risk associations for
  coronary heart disease 19,
    27–29, 31, 46, 48, 50
  sex differences 77
diastolic blood pressure 15
  risk associations for coronary heart
    disease 18, 20–23
  sex differences 13
diet 35
  Asian countries

China, stroke incidence and 63
  impact of changes 69–70
  Singapore 60
  cardiovascular disease prevention
    strategies 81
dilated cardiomyopathy 91
Disability Adjusted Life Years
  (DALYS) 74
Dubbo Study 44–45, 49, 50
  initial versus recurrent coronary
    disease 45–48
dyslipidemia 105
  role as risk factor in the elderly
    106–109
  see also cholesterol; lipid-lowering
    therapy

EAST (Emory Angioplasty versus
  Surgery) 132–133
electrocardiographic-gated MR
  imaging 93
electron beam computed tomography
  (EBCT) coronary heart disease
  screening 95–98
EPESE (Established Population for the
  Epidemiological Study of the
  Elderly) 107, 108, 122
estrogen therapy *see* hormone
  replacement therapy
European Atherosclerosis Society
  (EAS) 111
European Society of Cardiology
  (ESC) 111
European Society of Hypertension
  (ESH) 111
exercise *see* physical activity

family history of coronary heart
  disease 32
fibrinogen 32

FLARE study 102–103, 119
fluvastatin 101, 117–118
Framingham Risk Score 111
Framingham Study 10–35, 50, 106,
    108

gender differences *see* sex differences
glucose intolerance 16
    risk associations for coronary heart
        disease 19, 27
glucose metabolism
    age-related changes 16
    risk associations for coronary heart
        disease 19, 27–29
GUSTO–1 (Global Utilization of
    Streptokinase and Tissue
    Plasminogen Activator for
    Occluded Coronary Arteries) trial
    131, 133

heart failure 27, 91
    age-related incidence 11
hematocrit 32
high density lipoprotein (HDL)
    cholesterol 15
    coronary heart disease and 25, 44,
        46–47, 50, 111
        in the elderly 108–109
    sex differences 76, 77
Hisayama study *see* Japan
HMG CoA reductase inhibitors 117,
    134
    angiographic studies 101–102,
        119–120
    clinical endpoint studies 102
    coronary artery restenosis and
        102–103
    event-related trials 120
    metabolism 117–118

mode of action 118–119
    structure 117–118
    use in the elderly 120–125
Honolulu Heart Study 24, 106
hormone replacement therapy 73–74
    cardiovascular disease prevention
        strategies 83, 84–85
    coronary heart disease and 78–81
3-hydroxy–3-methylglutaric acid 118
hydroxymethylglutaryl coenzyme A
    reductase inhibitors *see* HMG CoA
    reductase inhibitors
hypercholesterolemia 45–46, 50, 107
    in older women 15, 16
    management of 26, 32, 34, 111,
        134
    see also cholesterol; lipid-lowering
        therapy
hyperglycemia 28, 32
hypertension 15
    China, stroke incidence and 62–63
    renovascular 92
    risk associations for coronary heart
        disease 21–23, 31–32, 43, 50
    see also antihypertensive drug
        therapy; blood pressure

India 61–62
insulin-dependent diabetes mellitus 28

Japan
    asymptomatic lacunar infarction,
        risk factors 66–67
    changes in elderly population 67–68
    cholesterol levels 67
    incidence of cardiovascular disease
        64, 65
    incidence of stroke 64, 65, 67–68
    mortality causes 57

KAPS (Kaiser Permanente Study)
106, 119

lacunar infarction, asymptomatic
66–67
left ventricular hypertrophy 17
risk associations for coronary heart
disease 29
life expectancy
sex differences 73, 76
women 74–75
lifestyle
impact of changes in Asian
countries 69–70
women 73, 84
see also alcohol consumption;
cigarette smoking; diet; physical
activity
Lipid Research Clinics Prevalence
Study 45
lipid-lowering therapy 25–26, 32, 35,
82, 101–103
absolute risk limitations as basis for
therapeutic decisions 111–112
angiographic studies 101–102,
119–120
clinical endpoint studies 102
coronary artery restenosis and
102–103
event-related trials 120
future prospects 124–125
in the elderly 50–51
cost-effectiveness analysis
134–138
evidence of benefit 109, 124
for primary prevention 109–111
trial inferences 49, 101
see also cardiovascular
interventions; HMG CoA
reductase inhibitors

lipids *see* cholesterol; triglycerides
lipoprotein(a) 46, 48, 50
lovastatin 101, 117–118, 119, 135–136
Lovastatin Restenosis Trial 102
low density lipoprotein (LDL)
cholesterol 15
Churchill phenomenon 107
reduction by HMG CoA reductase
inhibitors 101–102, 119
risk associations for coronary heart
disease 25–26, 43, 45–47, 49,
101

magnetic resonance angiography
(MRA) 92
arterial compliance estimation
93–94
atherosclerotic plaque
characterization 98
coronary anatomy and flow
evaluation 94–95
Malaysia 58, 59
menopause 73, 78
coronary heart disease and 78–81
see also hormone replacement
therapy
mevalonic acid 118
MONICA project 62, 64, 76
mortality
causes of death in Asian countries
56–63
changes in elderly Japanese
population 67–68
decline in industrialized nations
34–35, 73, 76
in women 74, 79
international differences 75–76
sex differences 77–78
Multiple Risk Factor Intervention
Trial 101

myocardial infarction 12, 26, 45,
    68–69, 91
    age-related incidence 11
    asymptomatic 12–13, 66–67, 78
    cholesterol levels and 121–122
    in Japan 64, 65
    in women 78
    lipid-lowering therapy and 134–135
    silent myocardial ischemia 68–69,
    78

National Cholesterol Education
    Program (NCEP), US 111, 135
National Heart Foundation, New
    Zealand 111
non-invasive vascular imaging 91–98
    arterial compliance estimation
    92–94
    atherosclerotic plaque
    characterization 98
    electron beam computed
    tomography 95–98
    magnetic resonance imaging of
    coronary anatomy and flow
    94–96
    vascular pathoanatomy
    identification 92
Nurses' Health Study 80

obesity 16–17
    Singapore 61
Okinawa study *see* Japan

passive smoking 77
percutaneous transluminal coronary
    angioplasty
    (PTCA) 69, 132–133
peripheral arterial disease, age-related
    incidence 11

Philippines 58
physical activity
    cardiovascular disease prevention
    strategies 81
    coronary heart disease risks and
    30–31, 77
    postmenopausal women 77
    see also sedentarism
Physicians' Health Study 109
pravastatin 49, 101, 117–118, 119,
    134–135
Premarin 78

REGRESS study 119
relative risk 112
renal arterial stenosis 92
renovascular hypertension 92
restenosis of coronary arteries 102–103
revascularization techniques,
    cost-effectiveness
    analysis 131–133
risk factors 9–10, 43, 76–77, 121–123
    age-related changes 13–18,
    121–122
    associations with coronary heart
    disease 18–32
    Japan
        asymptomatic lacunar infarction
        66–67
        changes in elderly population
        67–68
    risk profiles in the elderly 32–34
    sex differences 76–77
    see also individual risk factors
RITA (Randomized Intervention
    Treatment of Angina) study
    132–133

SAVE (Survival and Ventricular
    Enlargement) study 132

Scandinavian Simvastatin Survival
Study (4S) 49, 102, 110, 120, 124,
125, 134, 136
sedentarism
Singapore 61
see also physical activity
serum cholesterol *see* cholesterol
Seven Countries' Study 45
sex differences
cardiovascular disease mortality and
morbidity 77–78
coronary heart disease incidence
11–12
diastolic blood pressure 13
life expectancy 73, 76
risk factors 76–77
Sheffield tables 111–112
SHEP (Systolic Hypertension in the
Elderly Program) 23
SHIPS 102
silent myocardial ischemia 68–69, 78
simvastatin 101, 117–118
see also Scandinavian Simvastatin
Survival Study
Singapore 59–61
aging population 60
dietary changes 60
mortality causes 59–60
obesity 61
sedentarism 61
smoking 61
smoking *see* cigarette smoking
streptokinase 133
stroke
age-related incidence 11
Asian countries
as cause of death 56–63
changes in elderly population
67–68
China 62–63, 67–68
Japan 64, 65, 67–68

MONICA project 64
incidence in women 74
mortality
Asian countries 56–63
international differences 75–76
prevention strategies 85–87, 125
systolic hypertension and 23
see also cardiovascular diseases
sudden death 12
age-related incidence 11
systolic blood pressure
age-related changes 14–15, 76
risk associations for coronary heart
disease 18, 20–23

Thailand 58, 59
three-dimensional time-of-flight
MRA 92
tissue plasminogen activator (TPA) 133
tobacco smoking *see* cigarette smoking
triglycerides
in the elderly 109
risk associations for coronary heart
disease 25, 44, 46–47, 50

United States Preventive Services
Task Force 135

velocity-encoded cine MR imaging 94
very low density lipoprotein (VLDL)
cholesterol 15
vital capacity 19

weight *see* body weight
white blood cell count 32
Whitehall Study 109
women

cardiovascular disease prevention
   strategies 81–87
global cardiovascular disease
   burden 74–75, 84
see also hormone replacement
   therapy; menopause; sex
   differences

World Health Organization 75
   MONICA project 62, 64, 76
WOSCOPS (West of Scotland
   Coronary Study) 102, 109, 120,
   134, 135